Survivor's Guide

REVERSING CANCER

A JOURNEY FROM CANCER TO CURE

Understanding the Nature of Cancer
Restoring the Immune System
Destroying Cancer
Psychological Healing
Regeneration

Dr. Gerald H. Smith

Survivor's Guide To

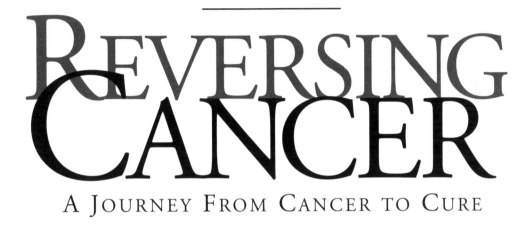

REVERSING CANCER

A JOURNEY FROM CANCER TO CURE

Disclaimer This book was written based on first hand experience dealing with a diagnosis of stage III ovarian cancer. This information is both general and specific as it relates to cancer. Neither myself, nor the publisher makes warranties, expressed or implied that this information is complete. The recommendations offered applied directly to my wife's situation and since every person is unique its contents may not apply to your circumstances. This information is intended as a general guide for cancer patients and not intended as medical advice, and we disclaim any liability resulting from its use. The treatment modalities used were those we deemed appropriate after medical consultations and our own research. Our opinions are presented as they related to our situation but neither myself, nor the publisher advocates any treatment modality. It is strongly advocated that each reader seek the advice of a qualified professional for medical problems, especially those involving cancer.

Dedication: Research represents a continuum of intelligent evolution. Many thousands of people have dedicated their professional careers to help solve the myriad of riddles that relate to the disease process. My thanks goes out to all those who have given their dedication and untiring effort to help conquer cancer. Special appreciation is offered to those mentors who taught me how to see the real problem behind the symptom. Finally, I would like to dedicate this book to my soul mate, who gave me the biggest challenge of my life-reversing cancer. The story that follows portrays the journey that enriched our lives beyond belief.

Edited By: Steve O'Neill

ICNR Publishing Company
303 Corporate Drive East
Langhorne, PA 19047
215-968-4324

Smith, Gerald H.
Reversing Cancer: A Survivor's Guide To
- Understanding the nature of cancer
- Restoring the immune system
- Psychological healing
- Destroying cancer
- Detoxification
- Regeneration
An integrated approach utilizing new technology
Includes bibliographical references and index.

Library of Congress Control Number:2004092511
ISBN 0-9617838-2-6

Survivor's Guide To

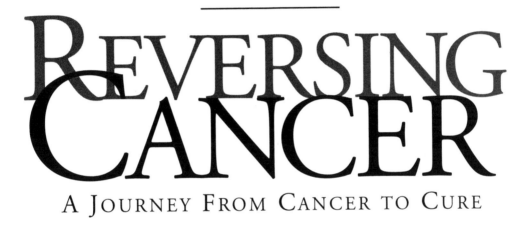

REVERSING CANCER

A JOURNEY FROM CANCER TO CURE

Understanding the Nature of Cancer
Restoring the Immune System
Destroying Cancer
Psychological Healing
Regeneration

Dr. Gerald H. Smith

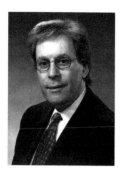

ABOUT THE AUTHOR

Doctor Gerald H. Smith graduated Temple University School of Dentistry in 1969 and completed a two-year tour of active duty as a captain in the U.S. Army Dental Corp. After practicing conventional dentistry for four years, Dr. Smith completed a two-year post-graduate orthodontic program in 1976.

Doctor Smith's broad base of post-graduate training has enabled him to integrate many health care specialties. He has accumulated an impressive list of credentials, which includes lecturing at Walter Reed Army Medical Center, National Academy of General Dentistry, Academy of Head, Neck and Facial Pain, Yonsei Memorial Hospital in Seoul Korea and dozens of guest lecture appearances at national and international symposia. He has memberships in and affiliations with a number of professional associations including the International Associations for Orthodontists and Academy of Head, Neck and Facial Pain. He has been an active member of the Holistic Dental Association since 1993, the president of the Holistic Dental Association and editor of their professional journal until 2005. He was also president of the Pennsylvania Craniomandibular Society.

Doctor Gerald Smith is a recognized international authority on craniomandibular somatic disorders with a focus on resolving chronic pain. He is author of two landmark textbooks for professionals, Cranial-Dental-Sacral Complex and Dental Orthogonal Radiographic Analysis. He has also written an important book for the layperson, *Headaches Aren't Forever*, and a newly published book on CD ROM, *Alternative Treatments For Conquering Chronic Pain*. Doctor Smith's thirty years of clinical research has identified several of the major missing links for successfully treating cancer and chronic pain.

In addition, Dr. Smith has published over thirty articles and contributed chapters to several professional books, developer of the Physiologic Adaptive Range Concept and a special dental x-ray analysis system. He holds two US Patents: a unique precision attachment for dental fixed bridgework and second patent for a flash adaptor to facilitate taking intraoral photographs. Doctor Smith is also president of the International Center For Nutritional Research, Inc. and he still maintains a private practice where he focuses his healing on chronic pain patients in Bucks County, Pennsylvania.

CONTENTS

FOREWORD

Reversing Cancer is the first hand account and personal journey taken by Sharon Smith and her husband Dr. Gerald Smith to put into remission a metastatic stage III ovarian cancer. This form of cancer using solely contemporary medicine's therapeutic modalities offers a five-year survival of only ten percent. The Smith's share their story so that past tragedies like the one involving the late comedian, Gilda Radner, who had succumbed to the same type of cancer, will become less prevalent.

Together they decided to integrate contemporary medicine with its known outcome and side effects with principles more extensively explored in complementary-alternative medicine (CAM). Doctor Smith developed an approach with primary principles he already knew while gathering new knowledge on their journey toward remission. These principles and their therapeutic modalities were again integrated to form a definitive protocol. This plan, as well as additional options for diagnosis and therapy, is clearly described for anyone diagnosed with any form of cancer and its associated risk of disablement or death.

Each principle is described in easy to understand language. It is apparent not only through existing data but by using common sense and intuition that they apply to restoring balance to body, mind and spirit. There is ancient wisdom and new evidence to show that this harmony has the potential to allow the body to better defend itself against cancer. Today, data supports the concept that eliminating processed foods from one's diet coupled with eating highly nutritious foods with appropriate herbal and vitamin supplements is advantageous in preventing and assisting one's body to better deal with cancerous cells. This approach allows for improved immune function and more available healing energy to cope with stressors.

Active infections decrease the body's ability to cope with stress and modify its immune response. Very little information is available in contemporary medical literature of the role dental infections play on health, immunity and potential for initiating cancer. Dental infections are also a major factor in cancer's ability to resist conventional and alternative treatment. The discussion of this problem is the most comprehensive and best explained that I have seen. Similarly, the discussion of chemotherapy, its side effects, and the need to prepare one's mind and body to deal with it more effectively is also well presented.

Each therapeutic modality discussed gives one the data upon which it is based or a source to reference this information. Also included is an extensive list of sources for the reader and physician to obtain each therapy. In addition, an informative and meaningful dialog offers expedient and efficient nutrient based alternatives to deal with the psychological aspects of the cancer crisis. These invaluable recommendations are based on more than twenty-five years of Dr. Smith's clinical experience, which also provides guidance for establishing nutrient dosage. I find it acceptable that Dr. Smith has referenced himself as one source for nutrients and herbs while also indicating other sources to investigate.

The ability to identify what therapy will be most beneficial for one's condition or illness has always been the aim of all those in the healing arts. Both contemporary and complementary-alternative medicine seeks to be evidenced based. Most clinicians would like to see data that is ideally controlled for bias and gives a clear percentage of responders to real therapy versus what is termed a placebo. Doctor Smith's approach to reversing cancer is based on real time medicine. His concepts weave the gentleness of the old time family physician, who took the time to listen and thoroughly examine his patients, with advanced technology that goes beyond the limitations of standard medical testing. The paradigm presented offers a sound foundation for medicine to build an integrated system to help win the War on Cancer.

If one intuitively or spiritually views the components of well-being as more holistic than the current emphasis, which is primarily aimed at destroying the cancer there is an alternative path. Evidence exists to show that changing the toxic environment in which the cancer lives takes away its support system to effect apoptosis or death of the cancer cell. Reversing the body's internal environment is in part the Smith's journey. If this philosophy and the existing data seem appropriate, I advise cancer patients to first work with their oncologist, surgeon, radiation therapist or any other primary/alternative health care provider. It would be advisable to be familiar with the principles of detoxification, nutritional support of the immune system, nutritional regeneration and the other healing aspects presented in this book before approaching the treating physician. The techniques offered are evidenced based and have been presented at medical conferences worldwide. The newer advanced technologies are non-invasive and have clinical verification and documented results. One must understand that most medical doctors have no more than three hours of nutrition during their medical training. This lack of knowledge accompanied by little to no clinical experience in the aforementioned approaches provides the basis for negative responses to alternative cancer therapies.

As a physician, I have treated many patients with chronic immune disorders in which complementary-alternative therapies have been efficacious. As a conventionally trained medical doctor who has made the transition and adopted an attitude of open-mindedness, I have gained much insight to this new way of thinking. It is important to look at the results of a therapeutic intervention regardless of whether or not one initially understands how this intervention works. The level of understanding of how the process may work becomes commensurate with one's increased database of knowledge of alternative concepts.

I commend the Smiths for not only their courage to directly face the prognosis but also for the trust in each other and risk for traveling the road less traveled. Based upon Dr. Smith's experience, research, wisdom and love, he offers us a unique gift of a guide for this unfamiliar road. I am optimistic that others will reap the benefit in what is contained in this book, which also gives us a new perspective to understand the many mysteries surrounding this dreaded disease.

Peter B. Himmel, M.D. Former instructor in Community Health at the Brown University School of Medicine, Former Adjunct Associate Professor In the Department of Applied Pharmaceutical Sciences, University of Rhode Island, Chief Consultant of the Himmel Health Center

INTRODUCTION On December 9, 2002 my wife was diagnosed with stage III ovarian cancer. She had scheduled surgery for what was believed to be fibroid tumors. At the pre-surgical examination and consultation visit my wife and I were told that if any complications should arise, an oncological surgeon would be called in to complete the hysterectomy procedure.

At 1:30 PM in the afternoon on December 9 my wife was taken down for her four-hour "routine" operation and I was off with two of our close friends to the surgical suite to await the routine post-surgical call and debriefing. During the seemingly endless wait, my son, my wife's sister, brother and our daughter joined me. At approximately 6:30 PM the gynecological surgeon called my son and me in for our "routine" debriefing. The look on the surgeon's face was not the usual congenial slight smile that she offered in previous encounters. We were told that the oncological surgeon was finishing up the surgery and that the diagnosis was ovarian CANCER. At that point I felt like I was hit in the back of the head with a two by four. My son and I broke into tears and cried uncontrollably. After ten to fifteen minutes we regained our composure and proceeded with the grim task of telling my family and friends. It was one of the most painful experiences I ever had.

The shock of the diagnosis was further heightened when I looked up the statistics about ovarian cancer. Each year approximately 25,000 women will be diagnosed with ovarian cancer and approximately 13,900 women will die of the disease. For the majority of women in whom the disease has spread beyond the ovary, the chance of living for five years after the diagnosis is between 14 and 20%. The pathology report stated that my wife had stage III undifferentiated serous type cancer with metastasis to several areas on the peritoneal lining in the abdominal cavity. Metastatic ovarian cancer spreads early by shedding malignant cells into the abdominal cavity. The cells implant on the lining of the abdominal cavity (peritoneum) and can grow on the surface of the liver, the fatty tissue attached to the stomach, small and large intestine (omentum), the bladder, and the diaphragm. Faced with these grim statistics and the aggressive nature of ovarian cancer, we sought a second opinion. Because time was of the essence, I solicited help from our neighbor, whose son had interned with the head of oncology at a prestigious teaching hospital.

Armed with the latest statistics, I asked the consulting oncologist the best treatment approach and the statistical success rates from such treatment. He replied that Taxol and Carboplatin were the gold standard in chemotherapy. He stated that of the initial group of ovarian cancer patients who had underwent the Taxol/Carboplatin protocol, 80% experienced success after a two-year period. He then told us that of the 80% who survived 50% had a relapse of the ovarian cancer. This group then underwent a second round of chemotherapy and at the end of a five-year period 35% survived. Percentage wise this translates to a 14% success rate. Anyone in business knows that it would not take long for any business to close its doors that showed a 14% successful sales record. Not even Arthur Anderson, who tried to cover-up Enron's losses, could have hidden this fiasco. In addition to this shocking news, there was absolutely no mention of the quality of life experienced by these patients during their treatment period. We left the consultation somewhat despondent.

My wife already had the surgery, and the surgical oncologist who removed the cancerous tumor told us that radiation therapy would not be effective in this type of cancer. Ultimately we were left with the only option medicine had to offer — chemotherapy. After reading the plethora of symptoms related to chemotherapy and my wife witnessing first hand the horrific side effects a close friend went through, she decided against this traditional approach. Her decision prompted concern from her surgical oncologist who urged my wife numerous times to start chemotherapy by the third week following surgery.

In 1997 my wife was treated for breast cancer and she succumbed to the fear tactics used by traditional medicine to undergo post-surgical radiation. After her lumpectomy the pathology report stated that a cancerous margin still remained and that a second surgical procedure would be necessary to remove it. During the two month interval between the initial lumpectomy and the second scheduled surgery, my wife treated herself twice a day with the Rife generator. The second pathology report stated that there were no cancerous cells present at the original site noted in the first pathology report. Medical confirmation of the disappearance of the cancer convinced us of the efficacy of Rife's discovery, in the 1930's, that cancer cells can be destroyed by frequencies. This positive news also motivated my wife to seek additional alternative treatments following post-radiation cancer therapy.

Our journey from the first bout with cancer to the present episode of ovarian cancer gave my wife the confidence to reject medicine's "gold standard" of chemotherapy and seek an intensive alternative approach. What follows is a compilation of the personal approach we chose with specific alternative treatments plus additional available therapies. It is our hope that this information will give cancer patients the knowledge and confidence to make more informed decisions.

The paradigm shift and innovative thought processes will challenge your belief system. That is why I wrote this book. By focusing on primary principles, *Reversing Cancer* offers the patient survival skills to help beat the disease:

- Detoxification of accumulated poisons;
- Change the internal environment of the body through high quality nutrition;
- Use of nutritional substances to boost the body's immune system;
- Employ innovative technology to destroy the existing cancer with minimal or no damage to the rest of the body; and
- To enhance the patient's mental well-being.

If one embraces these concepts and proceeds with an open mind, one will soon appreciate the great sacrifices made by researchers to uncover the origins of cancer and develop effective advanced treatments. One must also realize that sometimes surgery and other valid components of traditional medicine have to be integrated to conquer this disease.

The journey down the cancer treatment road is fraught with peril. Conventional medical treatment basically provides three primary avenues: surgery, radiation and chemotherapy. Selecting one or a combination of the three requires weighing the potential benefits and harm that can result. In our case, it was an easy decision. My wife's left ovary was the size of a small cantaloupe, and the right ovary was as big as a lemon. Our dilemma focused on the other two options. Since ovarian cancer is not sensitive to radiation, our options were quickly narrowed to one.

A cloud of skepticism surfaced after my wife identified the potential side effects of chemotherapy. Any kind of a quality of life faded with the horrible memories of what her close friend endured with metastatic breast cancer. My wife's friend stated that the chemotherapy took away a level of energy that never returned. She also said that, knowing what she did about the severe nausea and loss of energy, that she would never go through chemotherapy again. The clincher came from chemotherapy treatment received by her cousin, who also was diagnosed with stage III ovarian cancer. She was left with permanent paraesthesia of her hands and feet. The numbness precluded her from driving and because of her inability to feel she recently tripped and broke the head of her femur bone. The four months of post-surgical rehabilitation was arduous.

When compared to conventional medical treatment, alternative medicine presents a gigantic maze of philosophies, innovative technologies, magic potions, herbal compounds, vitamins, enzymes, homeopathic medicines, dietary regimes, detoxification programs and much more. If I had not been practicing alternative concepts since 1975 and had over twenty-five years of first hand clinical experience with many of the natural supplements, I would have been at a loss to make accurate, rational decisions.

My confidence in the capabilities of what alternative treatments can achieve was scientifically documented by conventional medical testing. I witnessed first hand the total reversal of a 73-year-old patient, who was in hospice waiting to die with severe congestive heart failure, with just vitamins alone. I also have information from a husband whose wife's breast cancer disappeared after having her mercury fillings removed, put on a nutritional program and used the Rife machine. The latter case was documented when the wife, who was hysterical from the initial biopsy report that her entire lumpectomy tissue sample, including two tumors and all surrounding tissue, was cancerous. To the amazement of the oncological surgeon, the biopsy report from the complete mastectomy showed all normal tissue. These and other dramatic results gave me the confidence to research my options and formulate a rational plan. The following pages represent the major treatment modalities, all nutritional supplements, and procedures we used. *An asterisk notes the therapies that were actually used.* As an added bonus, I have included other effective substances and approaches for your consideration.

There are no magic bullets. *A custom program must be designed for each patient, and the patient must be 100% committed.* It is important to select the supplements on the basis of patient compatibility. By being as thorough as possible, I believe the patient has the best chance for survival.

"The power of accurate observation is frequently called cynicism by those who don't have it."

George Bernard Shaw (1856-1950)

Section 1

UNDERSTANDING THE NATURE OF CANCER

The frightening truth is that the medical establishment has lost the *War on Cancer. Based on the American Cancer Society's 1999 statistics:* 1 in 2 American men will develop some form of cancer in their lifetime; 1 in 3 American women will develop some form of cancer in their lifetime; and In the 1930's the ratio was 3 out of one hundred developed cancer.

For countless millions, the cancer will not be put into remission or even contained by surgery, radiation and chemotherapy. Statistically 80% or four out of five ovarian cancer patients who receive one or a combination of the three types of therapy die within five years. Even more startling is the statement made by Dr. Hardin Jones, former physiology professor at the University of California department of Medical Physics. Dr. Hardin had been collecting worldwide data and studying cancer for more than 23 years. Hardin published his statistics in an article in Transactions, New York Academy of Sciences, series 2, vol. 18, n.3, pg. 322. Hardin stated that, "My studies have proved conclusively that untreated cancer victims actually live up to *four times longer than treated individuals.*"

The "War on Cancer" from 1972 to 1986 produced many casualties: "In thirteen years the National Cancer Institute spent 500 million dollars and tested 170,000 poisonous drugs for possible use in the fight against cancer. The results have been disappointing except in a few rare types of cancer.

Cancer research/technology may have become more sophisticated but the survival statistics have not improved. In reality, the possibility of even achieving a cure through standard methods has not advanced significantly since 1960. This fact is substantiated by the National Institute of Cancer's annual report, which stated that "Overall death rates increased through 1990, stabilized through 1994, and declined from 1994 through 1998 before becoming stable from 1998 through 2000. Interestingly, the International Classification of Disease (ICD) codes were originally developed to classify mortality data, such as from death certificates. In its expanded "clinical modification" (ICD-CM), it has come to be used for morbidity (illness and disease) data in a broad range of settings: inpatient and outpatient clinic records, physician offices, and other surveys. After reviewing the tenth revision of the ICD guidelines, it is this author's opinion that the stabilization of overall cancer death rates is due to the increased flexibility of coding mortality data and not the result of any medical advances.

Albert Einstein defined insanity as doing the same thing over and over again and expecting a different result! The insanity of conventional medicine is their primary focus on the villain with little or no attention being paid to the underlying cause. Medicine focuses on genetic engineering and destroying the cancer at all costs even if it means destroying the rest of the body. This myopic view is witnessed by their three principal treatments: Surgery cuts the mass out but fails to analyze the patient's underlying pathology (heavy metals, chemical burden, yeast or fungal infections, dental pathology, acid pH, liver toxicity, etc.). Radiation destroys cancer as well as the healthy tissue in its path. Radiologists never mention the need to analyze the patient's underlying pathology. Chemotherapy is a race between destroying the cancer before destroying the patient. Medicine's delivery system is "cafeteria style." Patients with a specific type of cancer get the exact same treatment with total disregard for their biological differences.

If medicine's methods were so successful there would be no need for alternative therapies, yet statistically more money is being spent by patients on alternative treatment each year than on conventional therapy. Moreover, if medicine has such a good success rate, there should be no need for intimidation and Gestapo type tactics to convince people to accept their treatment. *Frequently, parents of under-aged children with cancer who reject conventional chemotherapy are reported to Social Services and legally forced into treatment!*

WITNESSING SOFT-SELL THROUGH INTIMIDATION

I made plans to sleep at the hospital for the first two nights after the surgery. The day after surgery I witnessed the first of many "advertising campaigns." The well-orchestrated message was to sign my wife up for chemotherapy and start treatment no later than three weeks after the surgery. The rush to treatment was predicated on the aggressiveness of ovarian cancer. The presentation played out like a CIA brainwashing exercise with kinder, gentler performers. My wife just had extensive surgery. She was on powerful pain medications and totally drained mentally and emotionally. During the night before she was disturbed for blood specimens and vital signs. Then she was awakened at 7 o'clock in the morning for the first of many routine hospital procedures. Overlaid on these "normal" interruptions were several loud, piercing emergency code 2 announcements that were made on the public address system. It is amazing that any one can recuperate under these conditions. During the two days I spent with my wife, there were so many procedural interruptions that I was mentally and physically exhausted and I didn't even have the surgery or meds.

At the one-week post-surgery consultation, we were told that a three-week treatment hiatus would occur to allow my wife's body to heal from the original surgery. The doctor also informed us that successive treatments would take place at three-week intervals. Again the plan was to permit recuperation before the next round of toxic trauma was inflicted on her body. She was also given the option to participate in a controlled study that combined the latest in chemotherapeutic agents. Not once was there any discussion of her quality of life. There was no mentioned of dietary modifications or specific nutritional support in the form of vitamin therapy to be integrated into the plan. These concepts are just not in their vocabulary. Oncologists have no clue about the direct effect food plays on setting the stage and perpetuating cancer. One can also intelligently conclude that Dr. Otto Warburg's break-through discoveries on the causes of cancer were never mentioned in their oncology training.

At the two-week post-surgical consultation my wife, accompanied by her friend, met with the surgeon's nurse. The routine program was again presented, but this time my wife was given the grand list of chemotherapeutic side effects. Again it was stressed that chemotherapy was essential to destroy the remaining cancer cells and should be started no later than three weeks after surgery.

My wife took home and read with diligence the complete disclosure of chemotherapeutic side effects. Most people would not subject their pets to such harm and yet many willingly submit out of fear and ignorance. After serious consideration, my wife decided that she physically and mentally could not go through such traumatic episodes and decided to abandon conventional therapy.

At the three-week post-surgical consultation with the surgeon and immediate family members, a last ditch effort was made to sign my wife up for the program. Although skilled in his field, gracious in his bedside manner and truly concerned for my wife's welfare, he offered us no alternatives. In fact when asked about his feeling on alternative medicine, he replied I have no objections to whatever you do as long as it occurs after the chemotherapy. I politely stated that under such a scenario it would be an even more difficult task to restore a damaged immune system in the presence of any remaining cancer as opposed to just treating the cancer alone. No answer was forthcoming. This present day state-of-the-art medicine is looked upon as the gold standard but in reality falls far short of known scientific facts and the body's real needs. The ovarian cancer treatment success rate is only 14% to 20% in spite of the millions of dollars spent and years of research. Any major corporation whose annual report touted a 14% to 20% successful sales rate would be bankrupt.

REAL CAUSE OF CANCER

Cancer has only one prime cause. It is the replacement of normal oxygen respiration of the body's cells by an anaerobic (i.e., oxygen-deficient) cell respiration. — Dr. Otto Warburg-1931 Nobel Prize-Winner

The American Cancer Society (ACS) explains: "Cancer cells develop because of damage to DNA. This substance is in every cell and directs all its activities. Most of the time when DNA becomes damaged the body is able to repair it. In cancer cells, the damaged DNA is not repaired. People can inherit damaged DNA, which accounts for inherited cancers. Many times though, a person's DNA becomes damaged by exposure to something in the environment," a carcinogen like the chemicals in cigarette smoke.

In principle the ACS agrees that the causative factor is the damage to the cell's DNA. Unfortunately their priorities are misdirected causing them to go on an elusive chase. Medicine keeps searching for the best chemotherapeutic agents or other Sci-Fi remedies. No matter what their approach, their goal is still to attack the symptom rather than treat the factors that caused the DNA damage. By maintaining this illusive dream, a $200 billion industry is perpetuated worldwide. Because it will never find the cure, medicine will continue to perpetuate its myths about cancer.

THE NATURE OF CANCER CELLS

Doctor Warburg's discovery shows that cancer cells metabolize much differently than normal cells. Normal cells need oxygen. Cancer cells despise oxygen. In fact, oxygen therapy is a favorite among many of the alternative clinics; because, it is effective in killing cancer cells without damaging the rest of the body. Cancer metabolizes through a process of fermentation (production of lactic acid from the breakdown of sugar). It is a disease that is metabolic in origin, a disease that is linked with our utilization of "food." The metabolism of cancer cells is approximately 8 times greater than the metabolism of normal cells. Because of its high rate of metabolism, the cancer is constantly on the verge of starvation and thus constantly asks the body to feed it. When the food supply is cut off, the cancer begins to starve unless it can make the body produce sugar to feed itself. In its infinite wisdom, the body starts glycogenesis (gly-co-gen-esis), producing sugar from the breakdown of protein. Knowing that cancer needs sugar, does it make sense to feed it sugar? Does it make sense to have a high carbohydrate diet?

In part, food therapies have their successes because someone once saw the connection between sugar and cancer. There are many food therapies, but not a single one allows many foods high in carbohydrates and not a single one allows sugars, *BECAUSE SUGAR FEEDS CANCER.*

The presence of cancer signals the ultimate breakdown of the body's immune system. In reality, cancer is a generalized disease of the entire body. Every body has cancer cells during it's lifetime. The only difference is that when the immune system is functioning well the body destroys the cancer. Approaching the treatment of cancer should not be done in a haphazard manner. One must work closely with an alternative physician and biological dentist who can monitor treatment and test results. The key to successful treatment is to diagnose as many of the underlying factors that are contributing to the depression of the immune system. The following list of underlying factors provides a guide for evaluation and treatment. It is by no means all-inclusive but rather it provides a starting point from which to embark:

- Heavy metal toxicity (mercury, lead, cadmium, arsenic, aluminum, etc.)
- Chemical toxicity (pesticides, preservatives, fluoride, chlorine, cleaning solutions)
- Liver, kidney and intestinal toxicity
- Lymphatic drainage problems
- Poor Digestion (results in putrefaction or rotting of proteins)
- Constipation
- Dental infections present in root canalled teeth and old extraction sites
- Infections in tonsils or post surgical tonsil site
- Acid/base imbalance of the body
- Metabolic typing (fast or slow oxidizer; sympathetic or parasympathetic dominance)
- Nutritional deficiencies (high percentage of the population)
- Dietary intake of hydrogenated facts and refined foods
- Hormone imbalances (over or under-active thyroid, adrenal, thymus and pituitary glands)
- Quality of water ingested (PCB's, chlorine, fluoride, etc.)
- Quality of the immune system (T4 lymphocytes, natural killer cell cytotoxic activity, tumor suppressor gene antibodies, level of oncoprotein, plasma level of fat-soluble antioxidants, plasma levels of water-soluble antioxidants, lipid peroxidation, DNA repair enzymes, etc.)
- Quality of the blood (presence or absence of acid crystals, yeast, bacteria, clumping, fat deposits)
- Psychological component (biochemical components)
- Parasite infestation (intestinal, Lyme, Candida, giardia, liver fluke, etc.)
- Yeast, fungal and bacterial infections in organs
- Food sensitivities (stresses immune system)
- Level of distress in your life (moves, promotions, divorce, debt, etc.)

Not every person will have problems in all twenty-one of the above listed factors. Most cancer patients will however exhibit imbalances in at least ten of the above items. According to the clinical research of an internationally renowned cancer specialist, Josef M.

Issels, MD, (author of *Cancer: A Second Opinion*, 1999 Avery Publishing Group, N.Y.) a high percentage of patients with resistant cancers have infected root canalled teeth, infections in their jaw bones where teeth were removed and infections either in tonsils or the tissue surrounding the site of removal. As far back as the 1950s, it was Dr. Issels' clinical experience that when these dental issues were resolved, the resistant cancers responded to therapy. It is unfortunate that examination of these dental factors is not an integral part of the routine medical work-up for cancer patients. It is not this author's intent to provide a discourse on all twenty-one of the above topics but to provide essential information on pertinent selected topics, of great interest and benefit to most patients who have cancer.

HEAVY METAL TOXICITY

The most common heavy metals that most often affect our immune system are: mercury, cadmium, lead, aluminum and nickel.

Mercury Each year in the U.S. an estimated 40 tons of mercury are used to prepare mercury-amalgam dental restorations. Scientific studies have concluded that the amalgam is the source for more than two thirds of the mercury in our human population. Each amalgam, which is commonly called a "silver filling" by its installers, daily releases on the order of 10 micrograms of mercury into the body. This mercury either accumulates in the body or is excreted via urine and feces into our wastewater systems. After death, the accumulated mercury is released to the environment via either cremation or burial. Environmental mercury pollution is also caused by dentists who remove old fillings. Cutting out an amalgam/mercury filling releases colloidal mercury for which there are no commercially available filters to remove it from the water evacuated from the patient's mouth.

Heavy Metals and Chronic Diseases BY DR. DIETRICH KLINGHARDT, M.D., PHD In the late phase of the Roman Empire it was considered a privilege of the reigning aristocracy to drink out of lead cups and many of the water lines in the city of Rome were made out of lead pipes. It took several hundred years before the physicians of their time established the link between mental illness — affecting mostly the aristocracy — and the contamination of the drinking water with lead. In the 1700s the use of mercury for the treatment of both acute and chronic infections gained favor and again, it took decades before the neurotoxic and immunosuppressive effects of mercury were well documented within the medical community. Mozart died of mercury toxicity during a course of treatment for syphilis. Any pathologist in Vienna during that time period was familiar with the severe grayish discoloration of organs in those who died from mercury toxicity and other organ related destructive changes caused by mercury.

In the case of mercury, the therapeutic dilemma is most clear: mercury can be used to treat infections but — not unlike chemotherapy — also causes a different type of illness itself and may kill the patient. The same is true for most metals: small doses may have a therapeutic effect in the short term, life saving direction, but may also cause their own illness. Most metals have a very narrow therapeutic margin before their neurotoxic effects and in some cases carcinogenic effect, outweighs their benefits. Toxic metals may be fungicidal and bactericidal, maybe even virucidal, but many foreign invaders have the ability to adapt over time to a toxic metal environment in a way that stuns scientists and certainly outpaces the ability of the cells of a higher organism — like ours — to adapt in a similar way.

So in the long run, the situation looks different: toxic metals harm the cells of the body whereas the invading microorganisms can often thrive in a heavy metal environment. Research by Ludwig, Voll and others in Germany, by Omura and myself here in the US, showed that microorganisms tend to set up their housekeeping in those body compartments, which have the highest pollution with toxic metals. The body's own immune cells are incapacitated in those areas whereas the microorganisms multiply and thrive in an undisturbed way. The teeth, jawbone, Peyers patches (lymphatic tissue) in the gut wall, the ground system (connective tissue) and the autonomic ganglia are common sites of metal storage — where microorganisms thrive. Furthermore, those body areas also are vasoconstricted and hypoperfused (by blood, nutrients and oxygen), which fosters the growth of anaerobic germs, fungi and viruses.

The list of symptoms of mercury toxicity alone, published by DAMS (dental amalgam support group *www.amalgam.org*), includes virtually any illness known to humankind: chronic fatigue, depression and joint pains are the most common reported.

To keep it simple: mercury alone can mimic or cause any illness currently known or contribute to it.

Sheep Study Vimy, M.J., Y. Takahashi, and F.L. Lorscheider *Maternal-fetal distribution of mercury (203Hg) released from dental amalgam fillings.* Am. J. Physiol. 258 (Regulatory Integrative Comp. Physiol. 27): R939-R945 (1990).

ABSTRACT: In humans, the continuous release of Hg vapor from dental amalgam tooth restorations is markedly increased for prolonged periods after chewing. The present study establishes a time-course distribution for amalgam, Hg in body tissues of adult and fetal sheep. Under general anesthesia, five pregnant ewes had twelve occlusal amalgam fillings containing radioactive 203Hg placed in teeth at 112 days gestation. Blood, amniotic fluid, feces, and urine specimens were collected at 1-to-3 day intervals for 16 days. From days 16-140 after amalgam placement (16-41 days for fetal lambs), tissue specimens were analyzed for radioactivity, and total Hg concentrations were calculated. Results demonstrate that Hg from dental amalgam will appear in maternal and fetal blood and amniotic fluid within 2 days after placement of amalgam tooth restorations. Excretion of some of this Hg will also commence within 2 days. All tissues examined displayed Hg accumulation. Highest concentrations of Hg from amalgam in the adult occurred in kidney and liver, whereas in the fetus the highest amalgam Hg concentrations appeared in the liver and pituitary glands. The placenta progressively concentrated Hg as gestation advanced to term, and milk concentration of amalgam Hg postpartum provides a potential source of Hg exposure to the newborn. It is concluded that accumulation of amalgam Hg progresses in maternal and fetal tissues to a steady state with advancing gestation and is maintained.

Dental Mercury is Source of Two-Thirds of Mercury in Population Aposhian, H.V., D.C. Bruce, W. Alter, R.C. Dart, K.M. Hurlbut, M.M. Aposhian, "Urinary Mercury after Administration of 2, 3-dimercaptopropane-1-sulfonic acid: Correlation with Dental Amalgam Score" FASEB J. 6: 2472-2476; (1992).

ABSTRACT: There is a considerable controversy as to whether dental amalgams may have systemic health effects in humans because they liberate elemental mercury. Most such amalgams contain as much as 50% metallic mercury. To determine the influence of dental amalgams on the mercury body burden of humans, we have given volunteers, with and without amalgams in their mouth, the sodium salt of 2, 3-dimercaptopropane-1-sulfonic acid (DMPS), a chelating agent safely used in the Soviet Union and West Germany for a number of years. The diameters of dental amalgams of the subjects were determined to obtain the amalgam score. Administration of 300 mg DMPS by mouth increased the mean urinary mercury excretion of the amalgam group from 0.70 to 17.2 ug and that of the non amalgam group from 0.27 to 5.1 ug over a 9 hour period. Two-thirds of the mercury excreted in the urine of those with dental amalgams appears to be from the mercury vapor released from their amalgams. Linear regression analysis indicated a highly significant positive correlation between the mercury excreted in the urine 2 hours after DMPS administration and the dental amalgam scores. DMPS can be used to increase the urinary excretion of mercury and thus increase the significance and reliability of this measure of mercury exposure or burden, especially in cases of micro-mercurialism.

Flu and other inoculations use mercury as a preservative Thimerosal is a water-soluble, cream-colored crystalline powder. It is 49.6% mercury by weight. In the human body, Thimerosal is metabolized to ethyl mercury and thiosalicylate. The literature on Thimerosal metabolism and excretion is limited and old. Case reports have demonstrated toxicity after massive overdoses.

Toxicological information on the chief metabolite of Thimerosal, ethyl mercury, is extremely limited. During the recent controversy over the safety of Thimerosal in vaccines, toxicologists have assumed that the toxicity of ethyl mercury is equivalent to the toxicity of methyl mercury. The toxicity of methyl mercury is complex and depends on the type, level, and duration of exposure. The primary environmental exposure is through consumption of predator fish. A 6-ounce can of tuna fish contains an average of 17 micrograms of mercury. A pediatric dose of hepatitis B vaccine contains 12.5 micrograms.

The major toxicity of mercury is manifested in the central nervous system. Because mercury exerts such a tremendous influence on the entire body, it is in the cancer patients best interests to have it removed. Caution must be exercised in selecting a dentist who has a high skill level and knowledge regarding proper removal procedures including proper ventilation and evacuation devices to safely remove the mercury vapor during the removal process. Testing MUST also be done to select biocompatible dental materials (resins, cements, liners, crown materials, partial or full denture materials, etc.) that are going to be placed in the patient's mouth. A vitamin program to chelate the mercury out of the body MUST be part of the program. Equally important is to have intravenous infusions of glutathione, an excellent chelating substance, performed within 24 to 48 hours after each mercury removal session. This process helps reduce the body's burden of mercury.

Lead Lead in the body is dangerous because it interferes with normal body functions. It can change the way the blood-forming cells work, alter the way nerve cells signal each other, and disturb or destroy the way the brain makes connections for thinking.

Lead is a naturally occurring bluish-gray metal found in small amounts in the earth's crust. Lead can be found everywhere in our environment. Much of it comes from human activities including burning fossil fuels, mining, and manufacturing.

Lead has many different uses. Its most important use is in the production of some types of batteries. It is also used in the production of ammunition, in some kinds of metal products (such as sheet lead, solder, some brass and bronze products, and pipes), and in ceramic glazes. Some chemicals containing lead, such as tetraethyl lead and tetramethyl lead, were once used as gasoline additives to increase octane ratings. However, their use was phased out in the 1980's, and lead was banned in gasoline beginning January 1, 1996. Other chemicals containing lead are used in paint. The amount of lead added to paints and ceramic products, caulking, gasoline, and solder has also been reduced in recent years to minimize lead's harmful effects on people and animals. Lead used in ammunition, which is the largest non-battery end-use, has remained fairly constant in recent years. Lead is used in many types of medical equipment (radiation shields for protection against X-rays, electronic ceramic parts of ultrasound machines, intravenous pumps, fetal monitors, and surgical equipment). Lead is also used in scientific equipment (circuit boards for computers and other electronic circuitry) and military equipment (jet turbine engine blades, military tracking systems).

Most lead used by industry comes from mined ores (primary) or from recycled scrap metal or batteries (secondary). Human activities (such as the former use of "leaded" gasoline) have spread lead and substances that contain lead to all parts of the environment. For example, lead is in air, drinking water, rivers, lakes, oceans, dust, and soil. Lead is also in plants and animals that people may eat. Because of health concerns, lead from gasoline, paints and ceramic products, caulking, and pipe solder has been dramatically reduced in recent years.

What happens to lead when it enters the environment? Lead itself does not break down, but lead compounds are changed by sunlight, air, and water. When lead is released to the air, it may travel long distances before settling to the ground. Once lead falls onto soil, it usually sticks to soil particles. Movement of lead from soil into groundwater will depend on the type of lead compound and the characteristics of the soil. Much of the lead in inner-city soils comes from old houses painted with lead-based paint.

How might I be exposed to lead? *This Public Health Statement is the summary Chapter from the Toxicological Profile for Lead. It is one in a series of Public Health Statements about hazardous substances and their health effects. A shorter version, the ToxFAQs™, is also available. This information is important because this substance may harm you. The effects of exposure to any hazardous substance depend on the dose, the duration, how you are exposed, personal traits and habits, and whether other chemicals are present. For more information, you may call the ATSDR Information Center at 1-888-422-8737.*

People living near hazardous waste sites may be exposed to lead and chemicals that contain lead by breathing air, drinking water, eating foods, or swallowing or touching dust or dirt that contains lead. For people who do not live near hazardous waste sites, exposure to lead may occur in several ways: ▪ by eating foods or drinking water that contain lead, ▪ by spending time in areas where leaded paints have been used and are deteriorating, ▪ by working in jobs where lead is used, ▪ by using health-care products or folk remedies that contain lead, and ▪ by having hobbies in which lead may be used such as sculpturing (lead solder) and staining glass.

Foods such as fruits, vegetables, meats, grains, seafood, soft drinks, and wine may have lead in them. Cigarette smoke also contains small amounts of lead. Lead gets into food from water during cooking and into foods and beverages from dust that contains lead falling onto crops, from plants absorbing lead that is in the soil, and from dust that contains lead falling onto food during processing. Lead may also enter foods if they are put into improperly glazed pottery or ceramic dishes and from leaded-crystal glassware. Illegal whiskey from stills that contain lead-soldered parts (such as truck radiators) may also contain lead. The amount of lead found in canned foods decreased 87% from 1980 to 1988, which indicates that the chance of exposure to lead in canned food from lead-soldered containers has been greatly reduced. Lead may also be released from soldered joints in kettles used to boil water.

In general, very little lead is found in lakes, rivers, or groundwater used to supply the public with drinking water. More than 99% of all publicly supplied drinking water contains less than 0.005 parts of lead per million parts of water (ppm). However, the amount of lead taken into your body through drinking water can be higher in communities with acidic water supplies. Acidic water makes it easier for the lead found in pipes, leaded solder, and brass faucets to enter water. Public water treatment systems are now required to use control measures to make water less acidic. Sources of lead in drinking water include lead that can come out of lead pipes, faucets, and leaded solder used in plumbing. Plumbing that contains lead may be found in public drinking water systems, and in houses, apartment buildings, and public buildings that are more than twenty years old.

Breathing in or swallowing airborne dust and dirt containing lead is another source of exposure. In 1984, burning leaded gasoline was the single largest source of lead emissions. Very little lead in the air comes from gasoline now; because, EPA has banned its use in gasoline. Other sources of lead in the air include releases to the air from industries involved in iron and steel production, lead-acid-battery manufacturing, and non-ferrous (brass and bronze) foundries. Lead released into air may also come from burning solid lead-containing waste, windblown dust, volcanoes, exhaust from workroom air, burning or weathering of lead-painted surfaces, fumes from leaded gasoline and cigarette smoke.

Skin contact with dust and dirt containing lead occurs every day. Some cosmetics and hair dyes contain lead compounds. However, not much lead can get into the body through the skin.

In the home, adults and children may be exposed to lead if they take some types of home remedy medicines that contain lead compounds. Lead compounds are in some non-Western cosmetics, such as surma and kohl. Some types of hair colorants and dyes contain lead acetate. Read the labels on hair coloring products, use them with caution, and keep them away from children.

Air that contains lead particles usually exposes people at work. Exposure to lead occurs in many industries. People who work in lead smelting and refining industries, brass/bronze foundries, rubber products and plastics industries, soldering, steel welding and cutting operations, battery manufacturing plants, and lead compound manufacturing industries may be exposed to lead. Construction workers and people who work at municipal waste incinerators, pottery and ceramics operations, radiator repair shops, and other industries that use lead solder may also be exposed. Between 0.5 and 1.5 million workers are exposed to lead in the workplace. In California alone, more than 200,000 workers are exposed to lead. Families of workers may be exposed to higher levels of lead when workers bring home lead dust on their work clothes. You may also be exposed to lead in the home if you work with stained glass as a hobby, make lead fishing weights or ammunition, or if you are involved in home renovation that involves the removal of old lead-based paint.

How can lead affect my health? Lead can affect almost every organ and system in the body. The most sensitive is the central nervous system, particularly in children. Lead also damages kidneys and the reproductive system. The effects are the same whether it is breathed or swallowed.

At high levels, lead may decrease reaction time, cause weakness in fingers, wrists, or ankles, and possibly affect the memory. Lead may cause anemia, a disorder of the blood. It can also damage the male reproductive system. The connection between these effects and exposure to low levels of lead is uncertain.

How likely is lead to cause cancer? The Department of Health and Human Services has determined, based on studies in animals, that lead acetate and lead phosphate may be carcinogens. There is inadequate evidence to clearly determine lead's carcinogenicity in people.

How to lower one's exposure to lead The most important way families can lower exposures to lead is to know about the sources of lead in homes and avoid exposure to these sources. Some homes or day-care facilities may have more lead in them than others. Families who live in or visit these places may be exposed to higher amounts of lead. These include homes built before 1978 that may have been painted with lead-based paint. Federal government regulations require a person selling a home to tell the real estate agent or person buying the home of any known lead-based hazards on the property. Adding lead to paint is no longer allowed. But a house built before 1978, may have been painted with lead-based paint. This lead may still be on walls, floors, ceilings, and windowsills, or on the outside walls of the house. A previous owner may have scraped off the paint, but the paint chips and dust may still be in the yard soil. In some states, homeowners can have the paint in their homes tested for lead by their local health departments. Families can lower the possibility of children swallowing paint chips by not allowing their children to chew or mouth these painted surfaces and being sure they wash their hands often, especially before eating. Also a professional lead paint removal expert can remove and dispose of peeling or flaking paint or painted surfaces, and repaint the surface. Using heat guns or dry scrapping of old lead paint during home reconstruction and remodeling can be a substantial source of lead exposure to children. Surfaces should be tested before such activities, and professional home repair personnel should be consulted to make sure that safe procedures are used and removed materials and dust are contained in order to keep exposures to children to a minimum. Homeowners should not make these repairs, unless they consult with a professional to get the information they need to prevent the possibility of lead poisoning during or after the repairs.

Older homes that have plumbing with lead or lead solder may have higher amounts of lead in drinking water. You cannot see, taste, or smell lead in water, and boiling water will not get rid of lead. Running water for 15 to 30 seconds before drinking or cooking will get rid of lead that may leach out from the pipes. This is especially important if the water has not been used for a while, for example, overnight. Contact your local health department or water supplier to find out about testing water for lead.

If lead is used in the work place it can be brought home in the dust on hands and clothes. Lead dust is likely to be found in mines or smelters, where car batteries are made or recycled, where electric cable sheathing is manufactured, where fine crystal glass is produced, or where certain types of ceramic pottery are made. Pets can also bring lead into the home in dust or dirt on their fur or feet if they are exposed to high levels of lead in the soil.

Lead may be taken up in edible plants from the soil by the roots; therefore, home gardening may also contribute to exposure if the produce is grown in soils that have high lead concentrations. Certain hobbies and home or car repair activities like radiator repair can add lead to the home as well. These include soldering glass or metal, making bullets or slugs, or glazing pottery. Some non-Western "folk remedies" contains lead. Examples of these include greta and azarcon used to treat diarrhea.

Some paints and pigments that are used in cosmetics or hair coloring contain lead. Cosmetics that contain lead include surma and kohl, which are popular in certain Asian countries. Read the labels on hair coloring products, and keep hair dyes that contain lead acetate away from children. Do not allow children to touch hair that has been colored with lead-containing dyes or any surfaces that have come into contact with these dyes because lead compounds can rub off onto their hands and be transferred to their mouths.

Swallowing lead in house dust or soil creates an important exposure pathway for children. This problem can be reduced in a number of ways. Regular hand and face washing to remove lead dusts and soil, especially before meals, can lower the possibility that lead on the skin is accidentally swallowed while eating. Families can lower exposures to lead by regularly cleaning the home of dust and tracked in soil. Doormats can help lower the amount of soil that is tracked into the home; removing shoes before entering also helps. Planting grass and shrubs over bare soil areas in the yard can lower contact that children and pets may have with soil and the tracking of soil into the home.

Families whose members are exposed to lead dust at work can reduce contamination in children by showering and changing clothes before leaving work, and bagging soiled work clothes before they are brought into the home. Proper ventilation and cleaning — during and after hobby activities, home or auto repair activities, and hair coloring with products that contain lead will decrease the possibility of exposure.

It is important that children have proper nutrition and eat a balanced diet of foods that supply adequate amounts of vitamins and minerals, especially calcium and iron. Good nutrition lowers the amount of swallowed lead that passes to the bloodstream and also may lower some of the toxic effects of lead.

The level of a child's lead exposure can be measured with a blood test.

The following is a list of the major symptoms attributed to lead:

(Footnotes are at the end of each section.)

- Altered testicular functioning [24]
- Hypospermia (low sperm count) [3,5,19]
- Asthenospermia (sperm weakness) [3,5,20]
- Teratospermia (sperm abnormalities) [3,5,31]
- Erectile dysfunction, impotence [3,40]
- Decreased serum testosterone [3]
- Lead presence in seminal fluid [31]
- Pituitary effects [31]
- Sterility, infertility [5,31,35,39]
- Effects on ovaries [19]
- Decreased libido/sex drive [2,21,31]
- Impotence [31]

Kidneys

- Renal damage [2,3,5,13,14,21,23,24,28,30,34,39]
- Chronic lead nephropathy (kidney disease) [2,3,14,21,22,24,38]
- Death from nephritis (kidney inflammation) [29,30]
- Fanconi Syndrome [14]
- Gout [2,3,14]
- Renal hypertension [17]
- Increase in creatinine concentration [23]

Nervous system

- Encephalopathy (brain disease) [2,4,20,24,25,34]
- Cerebrovascular diseases, stroke, cerebral hemorrhage [2,27,28,29,30]
- Psychomotor impairment [13,34]
- Peripheral nervous system impairment (e.g. wrist-drop) [13,24,40]
- Slowed nerve conduction velocity (slowed reaction time) [2,34]
- Tremor [25,26,38,40]
- Paraesthesia, paralysis [25]

Cardiovascular and circulation

- Hypertension, elevated blood pressure [2,14,17,22,35,38,40]
- Increased systolic blood pressure in men [35]
- Cardio-toxic effects [14]
- Increased risk of cardiovascular disease [17]
- Coronary artery disease [2]
- Anemia; falling hemoglobin levels [2,3,5,13,24,35,38,39]
- Platelet dysfunction [2]
- Increased erythrocyte (red blood cell) protoporphyrin [35]
- Increased ALA in urine [34]
- Increased protoporphyrin in urine [34]

Intellectual and mental

- Depression [2,13,38]
- Anxiety [38]
- Personality changes [34]
- Death from violence, suicide, accidents [29]
- Impaired concentration [19,25,34,38]
- Deficits in short term memory [2,13,19,34,38]

Behavior

- Fatigue, muscular exhaustion [2,19,25,34,38]
- Sleep disturbance, insomnia [19]
- Irritability, agitation, restlessness, aggression [2,13,24,34,19]

Sensory

- Abnormalities in visuomotor coordination [2]
- Abnormalities in fine motor control [2]
- Deficits in visual acuity [2]
- Hearing loss [18,35,39]
- Somatosensory dysfunction (e.g. deficits in detection of vibration, changes in temperature) [2,23]

Digestive

- Effects on gastrointestinal tract [24]
- Loss of appetite [19,40]
- Nausea [19]
- Constipation, diarrhea [25,38]
- Abdominal pain, cramps [25,34,40]
- Weight loss, anorexia [25,38]

Bone, muscle and joint

- Bone marrow alterations [21]
- Myalgia (muscle pain) [25,38,40]
- Muscular weakness [34,38,39,40]
- Arthralgia (joint pain) [25,38,40]

Other

- Headaches [2,19,21,40]
- Decreased longevity [35,39]
- Adrenal dysfunction [38]
- Teeth with blue-black-lines near gum base [38,40]
- Pallor [40]
- Death [2,4,19,39]

Effects of lead from animal studies

- Impaired attention, learning and short-term memory in primates [12]
- Behavioral impairment; inflexibility in behavioral change in primates [12]
- Elevated blood pressure at moderate levels [17]
- Impaired immune system in new-borne of rats fed lead (greater susceptibility to asthma) [37]
- Altered response to stimulant drugs; attenuation of drug induced hyperactivity in rats [2]

Cadmium Cadmium appears to be the largest single contributor to autoimmune thyroid disease. It is a powerful, toxic metal, which seems to be at the center of the thyroid story.

Not only does cadmium appear to play a pivotal role in thyroid disease, it is a unique mineral. It is extremely toxic and has toxic biological effects at concentrations smaller than almost any commonly found mineral. Despite this toxicity, there is some evidence that cadmium is an essential nutrient with a biological function.

Cadmium depletes selenium in the body because selenium is essential for cadmium removal. Selenium atoms combine with cadmium atoms and leave the body via the bile system. When selenium is depleted by cadmium, there is less selenium to form the deiodinase enzymes, which convert T4 to T3, resulting in low T3 and hypothyroidism. Also there is less selenium to form glutathione peroxidase, one of the body's prime antioxidants. This results in greater levels of reactive oxygen species and hydrogen peroxide, which lead to an increased production of thyroid hormone and damage to the thyroid gland.

Cadmium and mercury toxicities (at high levels) will induce immediate hyperthyroidism. Vitamin E was shown to protect against cadmium toxicity and maintain T3 levels.

Sources of exposure: Air pollution, art supplies, bone meal, cigarette smoke, food (coffee, fruits, grains, and vegetables grown in cadmium-laden soil), meats (kidneys, liver, poultry, or refined foods), freshwater fish, fungicides, highway dusts, incinerators, mining, nickel-cadmium batteries, oxide dusts, paints, phosphate fertilizers, power plants, seafood (crab, flounder, mussels, oysters, scallops), sewage sludge, "softened" water, smelting plants, tobacco and tobacco smoke, and welding fumes.

Target tissues: Appetite and pain centers (in brain), brain, heart and blood vessels, kidneys, and lungs.

Signs and Symptoms: Anemia, dry and scaly skin, emphysema, fatigue, hair loss, heart disease, depressed immune system response, hypertension, joint pain, kidney stones or damage, liver dysfunction or damage, loss of appetite, loss of sense of smell, lung cancer, pain in the back and legs, and yellow teeth.

Aluminum Most people do not realize that aluminum is present in most underarm deodorants and toothpastes on the market. Use of these two products will result in adsorption into the body through the skin. Antacids are another source for aluminum. Underarm deodorant free of aluminum (LaCrystal deodorant stone) is available from the Allergy Relief Shop, Inc. 1-800-626-2810.

Sources of exposure: Aluminum cookware, aluminum foil, antacids, antiperspirants, baking powder (aluminum containing), buffered aspirin, canned acidic foods, food additives, lipstick, medications and drugs (anti-diarrheal agents, hemorrhoid medications, vaginal douches), processed cheese, "softened" water, and tap water.

Target tissues: Bones, brain, kidneys, muscles, liver, lungs, skin, reproductive organs and stomach (Agency for Toxic Substances and Diseases 1990).

Signs and Symptoms: High internal concentrations exhibit: colic, convulsions, dementia, esophagitis, gastroenteritis, kidney damage, liver dysfunction, loss of appetite, loss of balance, muscle pain, psychosis, shortness of breath, and weakness, excessive headaches, abnormal heart rhythm, depression, numbness of the hands and feet and blurred vision (Kilburn and Warshaw, 1993). Aluminum toxicity has been shown to produce impairment in choice reaction time, long-term memory, psychomotor speed, and recall in affected individuals as compared to controls (Wills and Savory 1985). Chronic aluminum exposure has contributed directly to hepatic failure, renal failure, and dementia (Arieff et al., 1979).

Among the clients in my practice, the highest aluminum exposure is most frequently due to the chronic consumption of aluminum-containing antacid products. Research shows that aluminum builds up in the body over time; thus, the health hazard to older people is greater.

D.R. McLaughlin, M.D., F.R.C.P.[c], professor of physiology and medicine and director of the Centre for Research in Neurodegenerative Diseases at the University of Toronto, states, "Concentrations of aluminum that are toxic to many biochemical processes are found in at least ten human neurological conditions." Recent studies suggest that aluminum contributes to neurological disorders such as Alzheimer's disease, Parkinson's disease, senile and presenile dementia, clumsiness of movements, staggering when walking, and inability to pronounce words properly. Behavioral difficulties among schoolchildren have also been correlated with elevated levels of aluminum and other neurotoxic heavy metals. (Needleman, H., M.D., Landrigan, P., M.D., *Raising Children Toxic Free – How to Keep Your Child Safe From Lead, Asbestos, Pesticides, and Other Environmental Hazards* (Farrar, Straus & Giroux Publishing, New York, NY, 1994) 38-39.)

Nickel A large body of scientific evidence supports the concept that nickel ion is carcinogenic. The hazard associated with a particular nickel compound or alloy largely relates to the propensity for the compound to release ionic nickel in the body. The evidence suggests that the relatively insoluble metallic nickel and nickel alloys are less likely to present a carcinogenic hazard than are the nickel compounds that tend to release proportionately more nickel ion (International Agency for Research on Cancer 1990).

Nickel compounds are known to be human carcinogens. This is based on evidence from studies in humans, including epidemiological and mechanistic information, which indicates a causal relationship between exposure to nickel compounds and human cancer.

Research conducted by David Eggleston, DDS of Long Beach California documented that placement of nickel alloy crowns in dental patients resulted in the lowering of the T4 lymphocytes within 30 days of placement. He also showed that thirty days after removal of the same nickel alloy crowns the T4 lymphocyte levels returned to their normal pre-placement levels. One of the major problems with metal alloys is the fact that when they are cast in a molten state to form crowns the alloy proportions are never the same. Even using the same batch of alloy does not insure exact proportions. This variation in metallic composition results in galvanic currents, which release metallic ions.

Sources of exposure: Appliances, buttons, ceramics, cocoa, cold-wave hair permanent, cooking utensils, cosmetics, coins, dental materials, food (chocolate, hydrogenated oils, nuts, food grown near industrial areas), hair spray, industrial waste, jewelry, medical implants, metal refineries, metal tools, nickel-cadmium batteries, orthodontic appliances, shampoo, solid-waste incinerators, stainless steel kitchen utensils, tap water, tobacco and tobacco smoke, water faucets and pipes, and zippers.

Target tissues: Areas of skin exposure, larynx (voice box), lungs, and nasal passages.

Signs and Symptoms: Apathy, blue-colored lips, cancer (especially lung, nasal, and larynx), contact dermatitis, diarrhea, fever, headaches, dizziness, gingivitis, insomnia, nausea, rapid heart rate, skin rashes (redness, itching, blisters), shortness of breath, stomatitis, and vomiting.

The greatest danger from chronic nickel exposure is lung, nasal, or larynx cancers, and gradual poisoning from accidental or chronic low-level exposure, the risk of which is greatest for those living near metal smelting plants, solid waste incinerators, or old nickel refineries.

Medical tests for heavy metal screening: Blood, urine, feces, hair, and fingernails. Two reliable sources for testing are:

Doctors Data:

> Phone: 1-800-323-2784 (USA & Canada)
>
> 1-630-377-8139 (Elsewhere)
>
> Fax: 1-630-587-7860
>
> e-mail: *inquiries@doctorsdata.com*

Great Smokies Diagnostic Laboratory

> Phone: 1-800-522-4762 (8am-8pm EST)
>
> Fax: 1-828-252-9303
>
> Web site: *www.gsdl.com*

Rethinking chlorinated tap water ARTICLE BY DR. ZOLTAN P. RONA MD MSC Most people never give it a thought. After all, public health officials keep confirming that chlorinated city tap water is safe for human consumption. Numerous scientific studies, however, report that chlorinated tap water is a skin irritant and can be associated with rashes like eczema. Chlorinated water can destroy polyunsaturated fatty acids and vitamin E in the body while generating toxins capable of free radical damage (oxidation). This might explain why supplementing the diet with essential fatty acids like flax seed oil, evening primrose oil, borage oil and antioxidants like vitamin E, selenium and others helps so many cases of eczema and dry skin.

Chlorinated water destroys much of the intestinal flora, the friendly bacteria that help in the digestion of food and protect the body from harmful pathogens. These bacteria also manufacture important vitamins like B12 and K. It is not uncommon for chronic digestive disorders as well as chronic skin conditions like acne, psoriasis, seborrhea and eczema to clear up or significantly improve by switching to unchlorinated drinking water and supplementing the diet with lactobacillus acidophilus and bifidus.

Chlorinated water contains chemical compounds called trihalomethanes which are carcinogens resulting from the combination of chlorine with organic compounds in water. These chemicals, also known as organochlorides, do not degrade completely and are generally stored in the fatty tissues of the body (breast, other fatty areas, mothers' milk, blood and semen). Organochlorides can cause mutations by altering DNA, suppress immune system function, and interfere with the natural controls of cell growth.

Chlorine has been documented to aggravate asthma, especially in those children who make frequent use of chlorinated swimming pools. Several studies also link chlorine and chlorinated by-products to a greater incidence of bladder, breast and bowel cancer as well as malignant melanoma. One study even links the use of chlorinated tap water to congenital cardiac anomalies.

Anything you can do to filter tap and shower water that eliminates or even minimizes chlorine would be helpful and possibly curative for some immune system problems. The use of filtration devices at the water source is increasingly popular and affordable. Discuss their use with a health care practitioner.

Dental Foci It is estimated that 70% of all medical illnesses are directly or indirectly caused by human intervention in the dental structures (teeth and jawbones). This includes: impacted teeth, infected root canalled teeth, new and recurrent decay around old fillings, cysts, bone infections in areas of previously extracted teeth, granulomas (areas of soft tissue that cannot heal) and areas of bone condensation (dense area due to calcium deposition) to osteitis (inflammation of bone) represent some of the more common factors.

Testing such areas requires injection of 1% procaine into the gum surrounding the suspected tooth. If there is a detectable improvement of symptoms far removed from the site of injection, it is a strong indication for the causal relationship. The improvement should last eight hours or more, according to current Neural Therapy teachings. However, there are exceptions to the rule with the improvement lasting only several hours. This testing procedure rarely produces false positive results and false negatives occur about 40% of the time.

Toxicity from dental restorative materials Dental amalgam fillings slowly leak mercury, tin, silver, copper and sometimes nickel. All of these metals have various degrees of toxicity. A fairly large mercury filling contains enough mercury to kill a child if given as a single dose!

The most common symptoms caused by amalgam fillings are:
- Chronic fatigue
- Tendency to chronic inflammatory changes — rheumatoid arthritis, phlebitis fibromyalgia, irritable bowel syndrome
- Chronic neurologic illnesses, especially when numbness is one of the primary symptoms
- Lowering of pain threshold

Allergy to dental materials used to restore teeth Having an allergic response to dental materials (gold alloys that include palladium, silver, platinum, iridium, mercury fillings, acrylic denture material which contains methyl methacrylate, chrome cobalt partial denture framework, nickel based crowns, composite resin crowns containing polyurethane) is a common cause of intractable pain, chronic fatigue, food allergies, chronic sinusitis and headaches.

Use of dental liners, that is, bases under permanent restorative filling materials can also be the causative agent for an allergic response. A new toxicity disorder discovered by

Dr. Omar M. Amin, Ph.D., Neurocutaneous Syndrome (NCS), linked components (ethyltoluene sulfonamide and zinc oxide) in the calcium hydroxide dental bases (Dycal, Life and Sealapex) as sources for the observed symptoms of NCS. The neurological aspects of NCS are characterized by pinprick and/or creeping, painful and irritating movement sensations, often interpreted as parasite movements subcutaneously or in various body tissues or cavities including the head. In the latter case, movement sensations are either unipolar or bipolar and may proceed horizontally or vertically. In no case was the movement sensation related to parasites, which were always found absent. Additional neurological symptoms include memory loss, brain fog, and lack of concentration and control of voluntary movements, pain, depleted energy and depressed immune system that may invite various opportunistic infections. In many cases, lesions are associated with swellings in the arms and legs. Blood vessels may also become enlarged and elevated, and the head may become hot and turn red and the gums and the teeth may turn gray.

Amin's study concluded, that the toxicity of the dental sealants (Dycal, Life and Sealapex) was well demonstrated in studies conducted in patients and controlled laboratory conditions by many workers.

For those patients who are having these toxic materials removed, it is recommended not to do more than two or three teeth per month. The patient is given a list of vitamins and other supplements to take during the procedure and for the following few weeks until symptoms are completely resolved. The list includes vitamins B12, B6, B5, E, C and folic acid, zinc, calcium, magnesium, omega 3 fish oil or linseed oil, amino acids, Acidofilus, Bifidus, Lactobacillus, digestive enzymes and selenium. After reaching a state of normalcy, the patient may still retain some sensitivity to moldy places. The sealants reported above are still in common use throughout the world. The "small" amounts continually leaching into the live tissues of the body promote a cumulative progressive damaging pathology over a long period of time. Dental practitioners should be aware of the adverse effects of these products and employ this knowledge to safeguard the well-being of their patients.

For those interested in reading the full text of Dr. Amin's article, Toxicity from dental sealants causing neurocutaneous syndrome (NCS), a dermatological and neurological disorder, it is available on the following web site: *www.holisticdental.org*

Electro galvanism When two dissimilar metals are present in the mouth with saliva (conductor), an electric current will flow. There will be a flow of electrons from one metal to the other and a flow of metal ions from one to the other. Any metal materials in the mouth such as gold crowns, chrome cobalt partial dentures, mercury fillings, titanium implants, etc. will set the stage for galvanic currents. In 1985, a research team (A. Knappworst, E. Gura, D. Fuhrmann and A Enginalev) revealed that when mercury fillings were in close proximity to gold crowns, the mercury release was ten times greater when compared to mercury fillings alone (pg. 132. *Mercury Poisoning from Dental Amalgam — a Hazard to Human Brain* by Patrick Stortebecker, MD, Ph.D. published in USA by Bio Probe, Orlando, FL).

Electro galvanism frequently is the cause for the following symptoms:

- Lack of concentration and memory
- Insomnia
- Psychological problems
- Tinnitus
- Vertigo
- Epilepsy
- Hearing loss
- Eye problems
- Mouth pain

Removing the mercury and other metals and replacing them with biocompatible non-metal restorations will resolve the galvanic issue.

All dental materials are potentially toxic with a broad individual variety of reactions. Mercury and tin are prime neuro-toxic substances. Mercury has the ability to destroy and or damage the transport fibers inside each nerve. The latest research from one of the top German toxicologists, Max Daunderer, MD, reveals that the entire jawbone (upper and lower) has become a toxic waste dump for the following substances:

- Pesticides
- Solvents (mostly present in lower jaw)
- Formaldehyde (mostly lower jaw)
- Amalgam (mercury, tin, copper and silver) — jawbone and maxillary sinus
- Palladium (from gold/palladium alloys) — mostly upper jawbone

Through biopsies, Daunderer found that virtually all inhaled toxins are stored in the jawbone in the areas adjacent to the root tips. Also of great interest is Daunderer's serial biopsies on malignant tumors in-patients that had amalgam fillings and found, predictably, amalgam in the tumor. The concentration is highest in the center of the tumor (malignant melanoma, brain cancer, bladder, stomach, colon and tongue cancer).

Root Canalled Teeth Boyd Haley, Ph.D., a researcher, at the University of Kentucky has estimated that 75% of root canalled teeth are infected. Another researcher, Hal Huggins, DDS, has shown that the toxins liberated by infected root canalled teeth are almost 1000 times more toxic than botulism. Botulism is the most toxic substance known. The following article provides an excellent overview of the potential hazards of infected teeth and mercury fillings.

CHRONIC DENTAL INFECTIONS AND TOXICITY

An Overview by Ilse Marie Issels, 2001 "In the western civilized world nearly everybody is confronted with dental problems some time in their life. In an understandable desire to preserve as many teeth as possible, to maintain the masticatory apparatus for health and cosmetic reasons, attempts are made to save teeth that are in fact lost. There is a widespread conviction that the sterile evacuation of the pulp of the root canal of the tooth followed by the refilling of the root canal is possible without any health risk. However, the dentinal canal does not end in just one opening that can be sealed. Instead, it resembles a tree with many branches that penetrate the tooth's body in all directions. Researchers have established that there is a lively metabolic interchange between the interior and exterior environment of the tooth, and that this two-way process takes place along many thousands of hyperfine, capillary canals joining the pulp cavity to the exterior surface of the tooth.

The structure of the root canal makes the elimination of all-dead pulp tissue, sterilization and filling of all the dentinal and capillary canals impossible. The microbes found within these dentinal and capillary canals of root canal treated teeth produce toxins that can no longer be evacuated into the mouth as the tooth is sealed. They are drained away through the cross-connections of the dentinal and capillary canals into the marrow of the jawbone. From there they are conveyed to the tonsils and the flow systems of the body reaching all cells and organs.

The most dangerous of the toxins found in root canal treated teeth are the thio-ethers, which are closely related to mustard gas and other poisonous gases.

These toxic substances seeping out of root canal filled teeth can damage enzymes of the body cells that are essential for their proper functioning. The resulting impairment of the body's regulatory and defense mechanisms can contribute to many immune disorders and chronic degenerative diseases, as well as cancer.

Moreover, many of the chemical imbalances found in patients are due to the reactions to toxic substances in the mouth. These include amalgam fillings that contain a high amount of mercury, non-precious metal crowns, beryllium, aluminum, and other metals found in fillings, bridges and braces.

Amalgam dental fillings contain from 48% to 55% mercury, 33% to 35 % silver and various amounts of copper, tin, zinc and other metals.

Mercury is a powerful poison that migrates in the human body for up to five years. It is more toxic than lead, cadmium and arsenic. Mercury, even in small amounts, can damage the brain, heart, lungs, liver, and kidneys, all endocrine glands, blood cells, enzymes and hormones, and suppress the immune functions.

Mercury vapor is continually released from dental amalgam fillings. Chewing, brushing, and drinking hot liquids can increase this process. Mercury vapor has been shown to settle in brain tissue. Mercury poison is linked to birth defects in newborns, as it can pass the placental membrane in pregnant women.

Bacteria in the mouth and intestinal tract mix with mercury to form methyl mercury, a substance 100 times more toxic. Mercury causes the normal intestinal flora to become mercury resistant and antibiotic resistant.

Saliva acts as an electrolyte when it mixes with amalgam fillings, to create a measurable electric current of 900 millivolts. This current overpowers the body's normal 450 millivolts, interferes with energy flow to the brain and is suspected as a catalyst in many illnesses.

Other alloys, such as nickel in the metal base of bridges and under porcelain crowns, have also been found to be detrimental to health. In predisposed patients, exposure to nickel can be a contributory factor in the development of cancer of the lungs, nasal passages and larynx.

The optimal strategy to prevent and fight non-responsive health conditions such as Rheumatoid Arthritis, Systemic Lupus, Lou Gehrig's disease, Chronic Fatigue Syndrome, Fibromyalgia, Sjoegren's Syndrome, Alzheimer's disease and last but not least cancer, calls for the elimination of all sizeable toxic substances."

Focus on Foci ARTICLE BY JOSEF ISSELS, MD The "focus" has been described as a chronic, abnormal, local change in the connective tissue, capable of producing the most varied distant effects beyond its immediate surroundings, and therefore in constant conflict with local and general defense (Pischinger and Kellner). By this definition, even a fully healed scar may sometimes act as a focus, spreading disease to distant parts of the body. But the foci we shall now examine will be confined to those of the teeth and tonsils — in my view, the most lethal of all foci.

The emphasis I place on the removal of devitalized teeth and chronically diseased tonsils is one of the better-known aspects of my work, but also one of the most criticized and misunderstood. I do not, for instance, recommend that healthy tonsils and teeth be removed from a healthy person. But I believe if they are diseased, they cause the body's natural resistance to be lowered, thus acting as an important contributory factor to tumor development. In these cases, I insist on their removal.

It is sometimes argued that to carry out such operations on seriously ill patients is unnecessarily cruel, even irrelevant. There are some unpleasant side effects, but in my opinion, the benefits — which I will describe — more than make up for any temporary discomfort. It is further argued that in the cancer patient, as much lymphatic tissue as possible should be preserved, and therefore tonsillectomy should not be carried out because even a diseased tonsil may retain some useful defense potential. I used to believe this was so. I do not any longer for reasons, which will be evident.

The beneficial results of tonsillectomy with cancer patients were first brought to my attention in 1953, and by chance. A tonsillectomy was performed on an incurable cancer patient in my clinic who had severe rheumatic pains and a long history of tonsillar disease.

The operation was done to relieve the woman's pain, but it was remarkably successful in other ways as well: general toxic symptoms disappeared and, most important of all, her pathologically rapid pulse rate was reduced. Many cancer patients have a high pulse rate, reaching 140 and even 160, and this always leads to a poor prognosis, but in the case of this woman, it was almost normalized. Soon her tumor began to regress, and ultimately she recovered from her cancer.

This unexpected but welcome result encouraged me to arrange for tonsillectomies on two further patients with tonsillar ailments, who also had therapy-resistant cardiovascular disorders and toxic symptoms. In these cases as well, following surgery, cardiovascular and many other symptoms virtually disappeared. A positive "re-tuning" of natural defense and a certain inhibition of tumor growth was also observed. This improved situation naturally allowed more time for active immunotherapy to work.

These early successes encouraged me to persevere with tonsillectomies. Before making them virtually obligatory in my clinic, forty percent of those who died there did so from heart attacks. Afterwards the figure dropped to five percent. This, I contend, is incontrovertible proof that tonsillogenic toxins find their way into the bloodstream and eventually can cause, for instance, a fatal myocardial disease. This is one reason why more people die from heart disease than from any other. In addition, my experience shows a direct connection between dental and tonsillar foci and many of the illnesses responsible for early debilitation and untimely invalidating.

It has long been generally accepted that head foci may give rise to almost all kinds of chronic, and certain acute diseases, such as-to mention a few-the manifold varieties of rheumatic and cardiovascular conditions. The removal of such foci is today a routine part in the conventional treatment of those diseases. However, the fact that head foci are also a contributory cause in the development of neoplasia, by lowering resistance, has received all too little acknowledgements.

The extent of the disease-provoking activity of a focus in distant parts of the body depends on whether the body is able to oppose the focus with its own defense mechanism. As long as the focal situation is kept under control by the local defense mechanism, no focus-induced remote effects will arise. On the other hand, distant effects will arise when the body's resistance has more or less broken down: control of head foci will then gradually collapse, and there will be consequential gradual increase in generalized focogenic intoxication. This will cause an inevitable deterioration of the body's defense power with a concomitant promotion of malignant growth.

Nearly everybody is confronted with dental problems at some time in their life, and even the most scrupulous dental care cannot guarantee dental health. Endogenous factors, such as prenatal damage to the embryonic dental tissue, as well as exogenous influences, such as malnutrition and toxins, must essentially be held responsible for the great number of dental diseases, be they a weak, susceptible gingival, or gum; or teeth which are malpositioned, barreled or impacted; or, worse of all, a disposition to decay.

Despite its porcelain-like surface, the crown enamel of the tooth is vulnerable to decay. Enamel defects develop especially in the grooves of the crown or on the adjacent surface of neighboring teeth, which are difficult to clean.

Decay is not painful so long as it is confined to this nerveless enamel layer. The onset of a toothache is the first noticeable sign that the decay has invaded the dentine body of the tooth, which, unlike the enamel, does have nerves. If this decay is allowed to continue, sooner or later the dentine will be completely penetrated, and the pulp inside the tooth will then become inflamed. As long as only the outer enamel and dentine are affected, the tooth can be preserved. But a tooth with an inflamed pulp can no longer be saved, and must be extracted without delay.

In an understandable desire to preserve as many teeth as possible, to maintain the masticatory apparatus and its functions, attempts are often made to save teeth, which are in fact lost. There is a widespread conviction that this can be done without risk by the sterile evacuation of the pulp, and then refilling the cavity. For decades, the erroneous belief was held that, after such treatment, the tooth is an isolated, lifeless thing, no longer involved in any of the body's processes. This assumption was originally based on the premise that the pulp cavity had only one orifice to the apex of the root below, and by filling this opening it was sealed. However, the dentinal canal does not end in just one opening; instead, it resembles a tree with many branches which penetrate the tooth's body in all directions.

Austrian researchers have exhaustively studied the finer details of the entire dental structure. They have established that there is a lively metabolic interchange between the interior and exterior milieu of the tooth, and that this two-way process takes place along many thousands of hyperfine, capillary canals joining the pulp cavity to the exterior surface of the tooth.

Very careful conservation measures may possibly seal off the vertical central-medial-tube of the dentinal canal, but it will never reach the lateral "twigs" branching off from this tube. Nor can it ever close off the innumerable capillary canals. Some protein will always remain in these secondary spaces. If this protein becomes infected, toxic catabolic products will be produced, and conveyed into the organism.

In 1960, it was established by W. Meyer (Goettingen) that within devitalized teeth the dentinal canals and dental capillaries contain large microbial colonies. The toxins produced by these microbes in a tooth with a root filling can no longer be evacuated into the mouth, but must be drained away through the cross-connections and unsealed branches of the dentinal and capillary canals into the marrow of the jawbone. From there, they are conveyed to the tonsils, and thus the flow systems of the body. In fact, the conservation treatment may literally convert a tooth into a toxin producing "factory".

A devitalized tooth is no longer able to perceive and control inflammatory processes even when suppuration has invaded the surrounding bone spaces of the tooth's socket; it rarely gives warning signals, for instance through pain, and therefore there is nothing to induce the patient to have this dangerous toxic foci removed. It then may be left to develop its devastating effect on the organism for decades or even for a lifetime.

When the inflammation spreads to the marrow of the tooth socket, it can cause osteomyelitis. Its further course is determined by whether and for how long the local defense is able to keep the focal disturbance under control.

If the body's local resistance is intact, a capsule of connective tissue known as the dental granuloma encloses the inflammation. This membranous cyst prevents its toxic contents from spreading into the organism. Radiographs of these teeth show granuloma cysts as more or less marked transparencies at the apex of the root. This type of tooth is called X-ray positive.

If the body's local resistance is weakened to such an extent that the inflammatory process cannot be encapsulated by the granuloma cyst, the toxins will be able to advance unhindered into the marrow spaces, the tonsils, and into the body. In this case, it is proof that — as stressed by Pischinger and Kellner — the organism has become largely incapable of reaction. Radiographs of these teeth as a rule show no transparencies, and are therefore called X-ray negative. In my cancer patients, I have found that such non-encapsulated foci — that is those who show X-ray negative — were particularly common, as one would expect from people whose body resistance has been lowered.

Today there is general agreement that dental foci should be cleared away, and it has become usual to diagnose them by X-ray. Unfortunately, only some of the dental foci can be discovered by this means. Encapsulated foci can be recognized only if large enough, and if not concealed by the tooth's shadow. And definite X-ray signs are much rarer in non-encapsulated osteomyelitic processes. It is therefore the most dangerous of all dental foci, which most frequently prove X-ray negative. Even with X-ray positive dental film, only those foci can be recognized which happen to be situated outside shadows. Since X-ray negative foci often escape treatment — and they are the ones the body has failed to resist effectively — they can continue to develop their destructive effects unhindered. My clinical experience has produced evidence of a causal connection between foci and tumor development, and in this respect, the results obtained with the aid of an infrared test are especially significant.

Any inflammatory disease focus creates on its corresponding skin surface a pathological increase of infrared emission; the higher the activity of the focus, the more pronounced it is. Using an infrared sensitive instrument (Schwamm's infra-red toposcope), the intensity of this emission can be continuously monitored and measured. Observation shows a close interrelation between the infrared emission of head foci and that of the neoplastic region.

That is, after treatment, a decrease in the infrared activity of dental foci was as a rule accompanied by a decrease in infrared emission over the tumor areas. From this it is clear that the advisable treatment for devitalized teeth is extraction.

But even this is not always enough. My experience has further shown that also living teeth may sometimes be so damaged that their pathogenic potential almost equals that of devitalized teeth. For instance, latent chronic pulpitis may arise in a tooth that appears outwardly healthy, thus having a focal effect.

The diagnosis and treatment of dental foci remains generally unsatisfactory. A survey conducted at my clinic found that, on admission, ninety-eight percent of the adult cancer patients had between two and ten dead teeth, each one a dangerous toxin producing "factory." Very often we are confronted with X-ray negative dead teeth, root remnants, and residual osteitis, which had not been diagnosed and therefore had not been removed.

Only total, thorough dental treatment will really succeed in giving the body's defense a chance. In addition to X-ray diagnosis, it is therefore necessary to use other diagnostic aids, such as infrared techniques, tests, to estimate tooth vitality and periosteal resistance, and other electrometric methods.

The diagnosis of foci in teeth had been greatly improved by electro-acupuncture. It is now possible to differentiate foci not only with regard to their type and position, but also to their virulence and pathogenic efficacy. The result of focus treatment can consequently be observed and improved, before, during, and after dentistry, to an extent never known before (Kramer).

If total treatment is to be performed, it is necessary to remove not only any devitalized teeth but also any hidden dental foci remaining in the jaw. Further, total removal of devitalized teeth and their roots must not be the end of the dentist's activities. Each alveolus — the tooth's socket in the jaw — should be radically cleared down to the healthy bone. In that way the development of the residual osteitis may be prevented. It is not only the tooth, which may be a focus, but also the adjacent tooth-fixing apparatus as well.

There are four different ways by which dental foci — and indeed all foci — can affect the organism and contribute to the development of secondary damages:

The "neural" way of affecting the organism When a focus develops anywhere in the transit tissues, the mesenchyme, the process is centripetally projected from the terminal neural organs around the irritated area, along the neural ducts, up to the corresponding control cells within the central nervous system. The irritation originating from a focus can, under certain conditions, trigger off the mechanism of a neural dystrophy — a slow degeneration — which may show itself in localized effects in other areas, but also in a generalized dystrophic disturbance.

In the 1950's it was shown that these manifestations are based on depolarizing processes in the affected neural cells, and in the corresponding tissues of the body's periphery (Fleckenstein and Ernsthausen). By elimination of the focus, the affected tissues may be repolarized. The most striking example of this repolarization is called "second-phenomenon."

Ferdinand Huneke, the founder of neural therapy whose remarkable contribution in this regard we shall look at in detail later, discovered over forty years ago that injection of a local anesthetic near a primary focus may immediately remove any symptoms of distant disease induced by the focus. This effect — the second-phenomenon — usually takes place only a few seconds after the anesthetic injection, and lasts for hours, days, or even for a lifetime. Naturally the improvement occurs only in those regions influenced by the injected focus. Nevertheless, the measure has therefore a remarkable diagnostic value as well.

Since neural therapy only neutralizes the neural effect of a focus, the focus itself must, of course, be removed after such treatment, in order to eliminate its latent toxic or allergenic action. Conversely, any focal surgery must be followed by desensitizing and neural-therapeutic measures.

The only exceptions to this rule are, for instance, featureless scars or other spots with no inflammatory change, which produce only neural distant effects without at the same time causing any toxic, microbial, or allergic secondary phenomena.

The "toxic-way" of affecting the organism The toxic activity of odontogenic foci is probably far more perilous for the organism than their neural effects. The mechanism of this distant toxic activity, as well as the characteristics of the toxic compounds involved, has been largely ascertained.

Odontogenic compounds are the gangrenous contents of an inflamed pulp cavity and its adjoining spaces. It consists of detritus and decaying, formerly vital substrates, which have been necrobiotically altered — commonly found in tissues destroyed by inflammation, liquefaction and microbial putrefaction. Thus there can be little doubt that they are genuine necrogenous toxins, including for instance autologous proteinic and higher-molecular fission products resulting from enzyme cleavage and other biogenic conversions.

Schug-Koesters, Hiller, Gaebelein and others of the University of Munich mainly clarified the identity and chemical structure of certain of the biogenic amines in the 1950's. Following similar findings in America, the German researcher Spreter von Kreudenstein further investigated the metabolic and exchange processes in solid dental structures. He showed that drugs injected intravenously were, four to five hours later, discernible within the intradental capillary ducts or even devitalized teeth, and in a concentration only slightly lower than in the blood.

Bartelstone (USA) and Djerassi (Bulgaria) have reported that endodental exchange may also take place in the opposite direction. If radio-iodine, I-131, is deposited in an evacuated pulp cavity which is then sealed off with a filling, the iodine will appear in the thyroid some twenty hours later, as can be demonstrated by taking a scintograph of the thyroid region. Similarly, dyes can be washed out of a sealed pulp cavity. Any substance produced by any of the structures in the oral cavity, teeth, gums, tonsils, will be drained by the lymphatic system and carried directly to the thyroid gland.

All these findings prove conclusively that within solid dental structures, there may proceed an unimpeded substantial interchange in either direction. Consequently, odontogenic toxins, wherever they may have been produced, are able to diffuse and circulate within the organism.

The German study group of Eger-Miehlke has investigated the pathogenic significance of these "endotoxins." They examined the changes in healthy experimental animals after injection of accurately defined, minimal quantities of the endotoxins from an odontogenous granuloma.

A single injection of a minimal dose seemed to develop a defense-activation effect. But after repeated injections, there was severe liver damage, and the animals died within weeks. Apart from the fatal liver damage, inflammatory and degenerative changes were found in all other organs, especially in the joints, muscles, and blood vessels. These results brought clear experimental proof for the first time that focogenic toxins act as causal agents for severe diseases in animals corresponding to similar chronic conditions in man.

The most dangerous of all odontogenous toxins are undoubtedly the thio-ethers, for instance dimethylsulfide. In a series of tests performed at my clinic, it was observed that patients with odontogenous and tonsillar foci had a heightened level of dimethylsulfide in their blood. After intensive treatment of the foci, this level returned to normal in just a few days.

Thio-ethers are closely related, both in their structure and their effect, to mustard gas and other poison gases used in the First World War. The extreme toxicity of the poison gases and thio-ethers can be attributed to the following properties:

- They are weakly basic, therefore "electro-negative", and thus they are deposited particularly in "electro-positive" cells such as those of the transit tissues as well as those of the defensive tissues.
- They are soluble in the lipids, and therefore have a pronounced tendency to enrich themselves in the lipoid-containing cellular structures, especially in mitochondria.
- These sub cellular organelles, attached to their lipoid membranes, contain the enzymatic structures responsible for the maintenance of aerobic metabolism — a precondition for full functioning power in all the body's cells and tissues. If these indispensable units are damaged, the most serious consequences will follow. Because they are the most vulnerable

cellular organelles, mitochondria are a favorite and almost exclusive target for thio-ethers. The action of thio-ethers is effected in three main ways:

- Since thio-ethers tend to combine with electro-positive metal ions and many bio-elements, which act as co-effectors or activators of numerous enzymes of absolutely vital importance, and as our present-day average diet is deficient in essential substrates such as vitamins and bio-metals, this deficiency is enhanced. Much of the daily intake of bio-metals, usually deposited in the fluids of a focally affected organism, will be made permanently ineffective; the more foci, the greater will become the deficiency.

- Thio-ethers are "partial" antigens, haptens, and thus they also tend to combine with the normal proteins in the body, "denaturizing" them. Such denatured proteins become "non-self" agents, which the body must deal with as such. The production of antibodies adapted to the situation will be provoked, and they will home in on the target antigens wherever they are. The process of "auto-aggression" will be set in motion: self-destruction of agents alien to the organism. Extensive structural cellular damage will result, increasing with age.

- The famous biologist, Otto Warburg, twice winner of the Nobel Prize, has shown that aerobically blocked cells — as caused by thio-ethers — will increase their anaerobic metabolism in an attempt to maintain their vigor. In doing so, they acquire the characteristics of malignant cells. Therefore, chemical agents capable of inactivating the aerobic process while increasing the anaerobic process are usually classed as carcinogenic compounds.

Druckrey (Heidelberg) found inter alia that transformation of a normal cell into a malignant cell requires a certain quantity of a carcinogen — the carcinogenic minimum dose. It does not matter whether this quantity is supplied in a single dose or in a number of smaller doses, because the toxic effects of each dose are stored, and accumulate without loss. The carcinogens held primarily responsible for the development of spontaneous cancer in man are those: Which inhibit the aerobiosis even in minimal quantities without at the same time immediately destroying the cell, and, which are constantly present in the organism in this minimal concentration of either endogenous or exogenous origin; they can therefore accumulate during the normal life expectancy gradually and unnoticeably until the total quantity necessary for malignization is reached.

There is hardly a carcinogen, which so completely fulfils these conditions, as do thio-ethers. Incessantly, from the moment the pulp is removed, hour by hour, year by year, minimal amounts of these most virulent of all the odontogenous toxins will be released into the circulation — minimal doses, but nevertheless sufficient to more or less totally paralyze the aerobic action of the cell.

The nervous system is thus doubly affected by focal intoxication. Firstly, by the increasing destruction of the neural ducts, which mediate between the control centers and the peripheral areas, thus sometimes initiating neurogenic dystrophy. And secondly, by the immediate intoxication of neural cells caused by the toxins spreading through the liquid vehicles of the flow systems, such as the blood and lymph. The more mitochondria a cell contains, the more it will be damaged by the enzyme-inhibiting effect of thio-ether compounds. Therefore it is the vital organs — the liver, nervous system, endocrine glands, heart, and reticuloendothelial system — whose cells may consist of up to one-fifth of mitochondria, that are primarily affected. Apart from disturbing regulatory control, odontogenous toxins will also cause additional damage almost throughout the body. Naturally, the higher the blood-level of focogenous toxins, the more severe will be their effect.

The close interlacing of the lymphatic and endocrine systems in the head, make it unavoidable that brain cells are more intensively toxified by the circulating focogenous agents and may suffer particularly heavy damage. The lymph ducts of the head region join Waldeyer's tonsillar ring, and if there is such congestion, waste fluids will be pressed through the porous base of the skull into the lymphatic spaces of the brain. Toxogenous changes, especially within autonomic nuclei, are regularly found in cancer patients, as verified in the 1930's by Muehlmann (USSR), and they may be a consequence of a life-long inhibition of cerebral aerobiosis due to focogenous intoxication.

The cerebral damage (diencephalosis) and the subsequent loss of vitality in cancer patients are accompanied by a number of other symptoms. The emission of hypothalamic energy impulses, recordable by a Voll's electro-acupuncture device, is reduced in patients with focal disease. The autonomic vigor is relaxed, creating "regulation rigidity" carcinomas tend to parasympathicotonic derailment; in sarcomas and systemic diseases, as a rule the opposite is found — sympathicotonic derailment (Regelsberger, Gratzl-Martin, Rilling et al). The diurnal, circadian regulation of the acid-base balance is lost (Sander). At the same time, there will exist a distinct inhibition of other diurnal control functions, for instance of blood sugar, cholesterol, and mineral metabolism, and many other metabolic parameters are greatly restricted (Hinsberg).

The lack of vigor and control efficiency is not, of course, without effect on the patient's psychic condition. Vegetative disorder is therefore generally accompanied by neurasthenic dystonia — characterized by the diminishing vitality and autonomic instability.

The "allergic" way of affecting the organism The toxic effects of thio-ethers overlap those caused by higher-molecular odontogenous toxins as already described. Antibodies are formed to fight these substances, eventually leading to the destructive processes in toxified cells. Since the kidneys excrete the organ-destroying antibodies or defense enzymes, they can be diagnosed in the urine by the Abderhalden test. In this way we can precisely deduce, in most cases, which organs have suffered secondary damage (Abderhalden, Dyckerhoff et all).

The extent of secondary lesions can also be demonstrated indirectly by vaccine treatment. Using desensitizing vaccines made from focogenous agents, reactions are caused in regions affected by distant focal effects, which may become evident in regional as well as general symptoms. It is thus clear that the development of cancer disease is, in more ways that one, closely linked with focal events.

The "bacterial" way of affecting the organism Bacterial dissemination from primary dental foci as a rule takes place with barely perceptible symptoms, and may be followed by the formation of "secondary foci" in other regions. These include, inter alia, foci in the paranasal sinuses, gall bladder, appendix, prostate, and renal pelvis.

Above all, bacterial dissemination tends to produce micro foci or micro thrombi in veins, and they in turn have a tendency to thrombosis or thrombophlebitis, possibly with concomitant embolism. Thrombophlebitis and thrombosis, so common in cancer patients, and generally regarded as resulting from disordered metabolism, are due not only to the dyscrasia of those patients, but also to the manifold effects of dental foci.

Shakow (Moscow), in collaboration with several clinics, has carried out an interesting investigation involving more the 1200 young pupils at a boarding school. Over a period of six years, it was seen that students with devitalized teeth had three times as many illnesses as those with healthy dentition. By removing devitalized teeth in these young patients, up to eighty percent of their illnesses were cured.

We have now seen how decisively the entire organism is affected by dental foci not properly treated, and what catastrophic results destruction of the pulp may entail. Dentists must, therefore, bear in mind that there is no root treatment, which does not inevitably produce foci.

The dentists' task is only secondarily cosmetic; primarily it must be preventive and curative. The over-riding consideration must not be conservation of the tooth but preservation of its vitality. If this is impossible, even the most beautiful crown must not delude us that the lifeless tooth beneath is anything other than a "corpse in a golden coffin", whose decomposition toxins slowly but surely are destroying the organism (Bircher-Benner).

Other foci in the jaw, for instance osteitis, cysts, foreign bodies, gingivitis, and malpositioned teeth may also develop focal effects. It goes without saying that these foci and centers of irritation must be removed. The dentist should always remember that he has a vital role to prevent the development of chronic illness and, most important of all, to decisively reduce the hazard of cancer.

Tonsillar foci. Chronically inflamed tonsils are primary head foci, which sometimes have an even more damaging effect on the organism as a whole than dental foci. They can participate in the development of chronic illness, including cancer, by the four ways already described for dental foci: by neural, toxic, allergic, and bacterial means. There are also similar connections between the development of cancer and tonsillar foci as there are between cancer and dental foci. For instance, after removing the tonsils, there is a decrease of infrared radiation over the tumor, and sometimes even a shrinking of the tumor.

The three tonsils in man, that is, the naso-pharyngeal tonsil, or adenoid, and the two tonsils proper, the palatine tonsils in the pockets between the anterior and posterior palatine arches in the back region of the mouth, together with other seemingly insignificant lymphoepithelial organs, form Waldeyer's tonsillar ring.

The tonsils are excretion organs by which the lymphocytes, microbes, toxin-laden lymph, and other matter, are discharged (Roeder). Even in healthy people, the tonsils may contain plugs — sometimes wrongly described as pus — which consist mainly of fatty acids, cholesterol, and other slag substances clearly characterizing them as excretion. The pale-colored plugs form in the shallow depressions on the tonsils' surface — the tonsillar crypts — and are expelled into the oral cavity and swallowed. The excretions of the tonsils may also contain dental toxins.

The tonsillar crypts have been described as the places where the physiologically obligatory bacterial flora is hatched. This flora colonizes the mucous membranes of the nose and throat and the other air passages. The tonsils also produce antibodies, and undesirable microbes and their toxins are rendered harmless. Thus they have an immunizing or detoxicating purpose and must be regarded as a functional analogue of the lymph organs of the intestinal mucous membrane, and, like the latter, as an important part of the body's defense system.

Healthy tonsils have a pale, pink, surface, and are normally almond or bean-sized. Not only functional demands and loads, but also to some extent by each individual's inherited constitution, determine their size and reaction capacity. With an inherited disposition to lymphatic diathesis, due mainly to heavy hereditary infection, there is regularly found a congenital enlargement or hyperplasia of the tonsils. This is always accompanied by an increased disposition to inflammatory reactions. Inflammatory reactions are also caused by their physiological function. A normally subliminal, and therefore symptom less tonsillitis, thus belongs to the "normal bodily state of man" (Leuscher).

Whenever large quantities of toxic and waste substances have to be excreted, the blood perfusion and inflammatory activity of the tonsils will increase. This state is often accompanied by painful swelling and reddening of the tonsils, and is described, depending on its subsequent course, as acute, sub-acute, or if occurring repeatedly, chronic tonsillitis.

I shall now concentrate on chronic, and especially on degenerative tonsillitis, because, under certain conditions, dangerous focal processes develop from it, which are of causal importance for the origin of all chronic illnesses, including cancer.

Although each case of chronic tonsillitis is due to the same mechanism, it is possible to distinguish between three different groups. The first group includes those chronic tonsillitis cases which arise in healthy tonsillar tissues capable of response, following frequent attacks of acute tonsillitis, or angina; they have been called upon to repeatedly react to infective irritation, and to excrete toxins. Each new attack leads to an increase in volume, perfusion, and activity. They are then in a high state of readiness for defense. But if such inflammations occur with increasing frequency, the tonsils gradually lose their reaction capacity and defensive power, and atrophy. Too much has been asked of them.

The second group includes those tonsillar foci, which develop under certain conditions from congenitally enlarged, or hyperplasic tonsils. This kind of hyperplasia can be so extensive that the fauces are completely obstructed. Unfortunately it is still common practice to reduce their size by partially lopping off these hyperplastic tonsils. The tonsils are thereby deprived of the shallow depressions — the crypts — so indispensable to their purpose; the excretory function cannot take place without an intact surface with open crypts. After a tonsillectomy lopping-off operation, the remaining crypts are always narrowed or closed by scar tissue, the substances to be excreted are cut off from their air supply (Voss), and are therefore un-aerobically decomposed with the formation of toxic decomposition products. It follows that lopping-off should not be performed. These tonsils should be totally removed, even if they are not yet causing any recognizable distant effects.

The third group of tonsillar foci, in cancer patients the most common, comprises the seemingly healthy, but small, congenitally underdeveloped and functionally deficient tonsils. A history of tonsillar symptoms is usually absent in these patients. Their tonsils are "unremarkable", but firmly fused with their base, and cannot easily be dislodged.

What these three main groups of chronic tonsillitis have in common is a focal-toxigenic effect progressively increasing with age, and a tendency sooner or later to atrophy. This process will be accelerated if there is an additional and continuous passive exposure to odontogenous (tooth related) toxins.

The close connection between teeth and tonsils was proven when it was observed that Indian ink injected into a sealed dental cavity appeared as spots on the tonsillar surface in about twenty to thirty minutes. These experiments showed that pathogenic substances from the jaw region, including toxins from devitalized teeth, are conducted to the lymphatic tonsillar ring, there to be detoxicated and excreted. Besides their "natural" physiological load, the tonsils are thus additionally exposed to continuous attack by odontogenous toxins provoked by the devitalization of teeth.

We have already seen how dangerous these dental toxins are. It is inevitable that they eventually have a severe effect on the active lymphoepithelial tonsillar tissue. So long as the cells destroyed by dental toxins can be regeneratively replaced, the functional capacity of the tonsils will not be seriously impaired. But if the destroyed lymphoepithelial tissue is increasingly replaced by inactive scar tissue — by tissue unable to execute its defense function — the excretion, detoxicating, and defense capacity of the tonsils will progressively diminish and eventually be extinguished.

With the loss of reactive lymphatic tissue, the tonsils lose their ability to give warning signs by inflammation; they no longer offer this usual signal for trouble. According to Kellner, this lack of symptoms signifies a definite inability to continue to further reaction. In such tonsils, the attacking toxins are no longer excreted; on the contrary, they are channeled into the organism via the vascular system.

It goes without saying that this development will take place far more quickly when less lymphoepithelial tissue is still present. In congenital tonsillar deficiency, there is, a priori, so little active tissue that its complete destruction can in certain cases be accomplished in a relatively short time. Normally developed, or hyperplastic tonsils if not lopped off, will withstand the dental infection considerably longer. But they too will sooner or later succumb.

The final stage of all three forms of chronic tonsillitis is therefore "atrophically degenerating tonsillitis." On medical examination, the findings here are small, atrophic tonsils, which show no sign of inflammation, but, unlike healthy tonsils, they cannot be dislodged by the surgeon's spatula. When removing them, they have to be dissected from their bed, so firmly fused are they to the surrounding tissue. Whereas with healthy tonsils the color of the anterior palatine arch does not differ from that of the oral mucous membrane. In atrophically degenerating tonsillitis there is a bluish discoloration of the palatine arch. The uvula is mostly gelatinously thickened. The tonsils themselves, however, may still appear externally healthy.

Even normal-sized or enlarged tonsils may already have extensive degenerative changes and consist mainly of hardened scar tissue, which of course is unable to neutralize toxins. There then follows the formation of usually quite latent and painless chronic tonsillar and retrotonsillar abscesses. Here we find the highly pathogenic beta-hemolytic streptococci of Group A — responsible for many chronic illnesses, and whose toxins spread through the organism and contribute to the development of secondary lesions, of resistance deficiency, and of the tumor milieu.

Apart from the directly allergenic and toxemic activity of these products, continuous toxic attack always leads to an alteration of the tonsillar (lymphoid) cells. Their proteinic structure is so altered that the organism is induced to form antibodies against these, its own, cells that have become foreign to it, antibodies which finally turn against healthy lymphocytes as well, and thus considerably weaken the lymphatic defense system of the whole organism.

With the decline of the active tonsillar tissue, its biological power is also exhausted. Active detoxification, toxicopexis, and excretion of toxic substances and wastes through the tonsils are no longer possible. In the tonsillar crypts, the physiologically essential simians are no longer hatched. Instead, dangerous pathogenic organisms are able to spread through the body because the immuno-activity of the tonsillar barrier is lost with the destruction of the lymphoepithelial tissue.

When the dental toxins are no longer neutralized and excreted, they will infiltrate even the last remnants of functioning tonsillar tissue and cause them to die. This creates high- and low-molecular necrotoxins, which, as we have already seen, are similar or identical to odontogenous toxins. Toxin formation is inevitably increased.

All these toxins no longer inactivated in the tonsillar ring or excreted, have to be conducted to other "vents" by way of the blood circulation. Toxemia and secondary lesions are increased, and the humoral milieu and the body's resistance deteriorate further. The process has become a deadly vicious circle.

Since degenerated and chronically inflamed tonsils are such dangerous toxigenic foci, like dead teeth and other dental foci, they must be removed. With previously lopped tonsils, there is also a clear case for tonsillectomy.

The focogenous toxicopathy caused by necrotic-atrophic tonsillitis is of course far more dangerous than the toxic-infectious effect of a hyper-reactive tonsillitis in childhood. And if the need for tonsillectomy is accepted in children, in cases of rheumatism and other comparatively harmless diseases, should it not be obeyed all the most urgently in tumor disease, especially as a causal connection between focal and tumor events can no longer be denied?

During more than twenty-five years of clinical experience, I have found that painful, enlarged tonsils and other symptoms of chronic tonsillitis were evident in less than one-third of my cancer patients. This suggested to me early on that the others might have silent tonsillar foci in the form of atrophically degenerating tonsils. In these patients with subjectively quite unremarkable, small, featureless tonsils, I examined their case histories, and searched for silent tonsillar foci with the aid of the infrared toposcope, the electrodermatometer, and other methods. These observations showed that, although most of them had never suffered from tonsillitis, there were clear findings of a tonsillogenic focal toxicosis. Whenever this was compatible with the condition of the patient tonsillectomy was performed.

The findings in these healthy-looking tonsils were incomparably more serious than even those in the obviously diseased tonsils removed in usual ear-nose-and-throat practice. The tonsillar capsule always proved to show callous thickening, and was so firmly adherent that the tonsils could only be dissected out. In about five percent of the patients there were fairly large peritonsillary or retrotonsillary abscesses, which had caused no symptoms. Far more frequently there were several abscesses as well as cysts often the size of cherries, full of liquid or condensed pus. The tonsillar tissue was spongy, slushy, and had a putrid smell. Histological examination of these tonsils always showed severe degenerative changes, and in the majority of cases, a complete atrophy of lymphoepithelial tissue. All these "featureless", clinically unremarkable, small tonsils proved without exception to be foci of the most dangerous kind which, like the silent dental foci, had probably been present and unrecognized for years or even decades.

These pronounced positive effects of tonsillectomy make it mandatory to always follow dentistry with treatment of the tonsils. In every tonsillectomy performed in my clinic subsequently, we found through biopsy severe or very severe destructive tonsillar processes with more or less virulent tonsillogenic focal toxicosis. The flourishing of patients after tonsillectomy is impressive and has been demonstrated to my clinical satisfaction again and again.

Toxins constantly circulating in the blood in degenerative tonsillitis cause a permanent spasm of the blood capillaries, seen outwardly in the poorly perfused, pallid skin of many cancer patients. After tonsillectomy and the consequent elimination of the toxins and their neural effect, there was frequently an immediate improvement of the circulation and a simultaneous improvement in the general condition of the organism.

As already mentioned, before I began paying special attention to the tonsils, I lost many incurable patients, not as a result of cancer, but through acute cardio circulatory failure. After introducing tonsillectomy, such deaths became much less frequent.

Toxic circulatory death, however, is only one of the many dangers constantly threatening the life of the chronically sick. Phlebitis, thrombosis, embolism, pneumonia, pleurisy, and cystitis all too often complicate the course of treatment. In my experience, these, too, became noticeably less frequent with the introduction of routine tonsillectomy.

Another observation, one I believe very important for cancer treatment, is that often following tonsillectomy, in a large proportion of patients, I have found that the tongue, not coated before the tonsillectomy, later has a marked yellowish, brownish, or blackish coating. Experience shows that the canalizing activity of the intestinal mucous membranes is indicated by the surface condition or coating of the tongue. A change in this coating suggests that a previously blocked "gut filter" has been opened, leading to the conclusion that tonsillar foci also disturb the detoxicating and excretory activity of the gut. Restitution of this function is of crucial importance in the treatment of cancer because this route excretes the largest proportion of the necrogenous toxins, which develop during tumor solution.

The widespread opinion that degeneratively destroyed tonsils may still be of importance for cancer patients as detoxicating and excretory organs and must therefore be preserved at all cost has, in my experience, been quite clearly refuted. Anyone, having seen the degenerative destruction in the tonsillar tissue of cancer patients, will be convinced that, on the contrary, these tonsils have contributed in potentiating the virulence of the tumor milieu and the defense deficiency. Tonsillectomy must be followed by desensitization with vaccines obtained from dental and tonsillar foci. Neural treatment of the tonsillar bed concludes this treatment.

Many clinicians have reported the increased tendency towards thrombosis in cancer patients. It can be assumed there is a causal connection between the two diseases. My experience is that this tendency is reduced by treatment of the head foci. I have treated cancer patients who were being given anticoagulants permanently because of their thrombosis; after treatment of the head foci, as a rule, they were able to discontinue these drugs.

In some cancer patients there is a secondary finding of therapy-resistant hypertension. Here too, following treatment of the head foci, the blood pressure generally returns to normal.

The growth of the tumor itself is very often distinctly slowed down by focus treatment. Now and then tumor development stops altogether, and sometimes even regresses. The head foci therefore seem not only to contribute to the development of secondary lesions, to the origin of cancer disease, but also to exert a direct influence on tumor growth by stimulating it. Many tumors seem to respond to immuno-therapy only when foci have been removed. The subsequent improvement in the body's defenses clearly shows itself in the response to immunizing vaccines.

Nevertheless, my own unhappy experience shows that with cancer patients, foci treatment has generally been left to a very late state. In the vast majority of the patients I have treated it is quite clear that foci treatment should have been carried out years before — and certainly long before the manifestation of the tumors. That this was not done is a sad reminder that far too many doctors and dentists fail to recognize a fundamental truism: untreated foci can be linked to the development of cancer.

PARASITES

Statistics show that over one billion people worldwide are afflicted with one or more parasites. Parasitic infections are usually associated with third world countries; however, the United States is witnessing an increased prevalence of parasite-related problems. In 1976 a nation-wide survey conducted by public health and private laboratories revealed that stool samples showed an infestation rate of 15.6%. Today it is estimated that infestation percentages are at 30%.

Most Common Clinical Parasite Symptoms The most classic of all symptoms involve the stomach and intestinal tract and include such episodes as recurrent diarrhea, alternating diarrhea and constipation, stomach bloating, intestinal gas, abdominal pain or cramping and nausea. General weakness or chronic fatigue not alleviated by extended periods of rest. Other common symptoms are weight loss or gain, intestinal poisoning, dysentery and perianal or perineal (area surrounding the thighs and pelvis) itching.

The poisons released by parasites can produce symptoms anywhere in the body. These toxins place another heavy burden on the liver, which is already overloaded by medications, chemicalized foods, leaked mercury from dental fillings, chemicals from deodorants, skincare products, shampoos, fluorides from toothpastes and our contaminated environment.

Common clinical indicators that parasites may be present are heavy mucus in the body resulting from parasitic mucous secretions. This mucous coating may prevent the absorption and utilization of nutrients from the intestinal tract. The presence of acne or other dermatologic problems, allergies, arthritis, headaches or even postnasal drip that does not resolve are potential parasitic symptoms. Furthermore, patients may develop sugar cravings and a ravenous appetite.

Medical doctors often misdiagnose parasitic infestations. This is especially true in patients with an absence of gastrointestinal symptoms but still present the associated symptoms.

Four Primary Classes of Parasites There are approximately 3,200 different species of parasites, which can be dived into four main groups:

- Tapeworms: they generally inhabit the intestinal tract. The most common varieties are the beef and pork tapeworms. Tapeworms go through three distinct stages of development in their life cycle.
- Roundworms: this group may inhabit the intestinal tract or may migrate into various organs (liver, lungs, pancreas, heart, or just live in body cavities). The common varieties are true roundworms or threadworms. Roundworms go through three distinct stages of development in their life cycle.
- Protozoa: Most protozoa are single-celled microscopic parasites that migrate through the blood stream to all parts of the body. Common forms are Guardia (most common one in the United States) and endameba histolytica, which result from contaminated water, food, handling pets or animals, changing diapers, swimming pools and other water recreation activities.
- Flukes: These parasites generally travel through the tissues and settle in the liver, kidneys, lungs or intestinal tract. Flukes are generally spread via contaminated water, nuts, vegetables and fresh water fish. In recent years, flukes have become much more prevalent in lakes, ponds and streams through out the United States.

Parasitic Cleansing Program To be truly effective any anti-parasite program for tapeworms and round worms must treat the three stages of development for these two groups. The protocol must provide separate phases to eliminate the adults and then successive generations of grubs and larvae before they mature.

Based on the treatment of thousands of patients with parasites, "Doc" Wheelwright discovered that a fifteen-day treatment cycle was the most effective schedule. Each 15-day cycle is repeated 4-6 times for a total of 60-90 days. Each 15-day cycle consists of taking the appropriate Systemic Formula product for ten consecutive days and then stopping for five days.

Each 15-day cycle is 10 days on plus 5 days off. This schedule must be repeated a minimum of 4 times, a total of 60 days, to insure success. In some cases 6 cycles, 90 days, may be required to resolve the parasite problem. Shortcutting treatment, that is less than 60 days, may result in more harm since this approach will offer only temporary relief from symptoms. The parasite problem will not be totally resolved, and the symptoms will reappear when the next generation of parasites mature to the adult stage.

Treatment Warnings: Abandoning the anti-parasitic program mid-schedule could be dangerous to your health. Patients must make the commitment to complete, prior to starting the program: minimum of 4 cycles (4 fifteen day cycles for tapeworms and roundworms) that is 60 days.

The necessity of staying the treatment course especially with tapeworms, known as the mother of all parasites, is based on the fact that they excrete a chemical into the intestinal tract, which inhibits the hatching of their eggs while they are still alive. This is the reason that there is usually only one adult tapeworm in the intestine at a time. Stopping treatment before the 60 day period will allow numerous eggs to hatch in the intestines. If these eggs reach adulthood, the body will be over run with parasites and potentially present a life-threatening situation.

Caution: An anti-parasitic program is NOT recommended for pregnant or nursing women or children under the age of six, or ages eight for the treatment of tapeworms with Systemic Formula VRM1.

Treatment of Parasites Systemic Formulas provides a convenient system for treating the four primary groups of parasites. Through the clinical research of A.S. Wheelwright, Systemic Formulas has developed herbal preparations that are just as effective as pharmaceutical agents but with much less side effects. The following supplements are designed for each of the four groups:

- Tapeworms: VRM1
- Roundworms: VRM2
- Protozoa (Amoeba, Guardia): VRM3 with WO (China Healing Oil)
- Flukes: VRM4 with WO (China Healing Oil)

It should be noted that the Systemic Formula VRM1 works for certain larger roundworms (nematodes). Also that VRM4 with WO (China Healing Oil) works for amoebas in certain cases.

Treatment with these anti-parasitic herbal formulas must be done in conjunction with your health care practitioner. These formulas are not available from health food stores.

Fluke Worms and cancer An independent research scientist, Hulda Clark, presented her controversial cancer theories in her book "The Cure For All Cancers". This overview is a synopsis of her book. Although Clark claims that all cancers are the result of parasitic infestations, my clinical experience has shown that in most cases there are multiple causes for cancer. It behooves one to seek out an alternative physician who has a broad understanding of heavy metals, chemical toxicities, parasites, dental foci, nutritional factors and the wisdom to refer you to the appropriate practitioner who can assess structural imbalances (osteopath or chiropractor), biologic dentist (jawbone and root canal infections, mercury poisoning, dental material incompatibilities), oncological surgeon (specialize in cancer), psychological component, energy imbalances (acupuncturist) and any other qualified practitioner that may benefit you. One of the keys to successful treatment is an integrated approach of all health care fields to resolve the underlying causes.

Hulda Clark states that the cause of cancers is a single parasite, the human intestinal fluke. The theory is if you kill the parasite that the cancer stops immediately and the tissue becomes normal. How can a simple intestinal fluke cause such destruction and where does this parasite come from? This fluke typically lives inside one's intestine where it does little harm other than causing irritable bowel syndrome or colitis. If however this fluke invades other organs of the body it does a great deal of harm. According to Hulda Clark the presence of propyl alcohol sets the stage for cancer to develop.

The intestinal fluke is a parasite that is about 3/4 of an inch long and is flat as a leaf. Like most parasites it invades a host and then lays it eggs, which are typically passed out of the host with a bowel movement. The adult intestinal fluke however stays tightly stuck to the walls of the intestines.

Tiny lesions in our intestines allow some of the microscopic eggs to get into the blood stream and hatch. The microscopic hatchlings are called miracidia and represent the second stage in the life cycle of this parasite. These miracidia are mobile and will migrate to the liver. Under normal circumstances in healthy people these miracidia are killed when they reach the liver. But in the presence of propyl alcohol the liver is unable to kill this second stage parasite and the miracidia begin to make redia, the third stage of the parasite.

The parasite is laying eggs and producing millions of redia in your body. Smoker's lungs, breasts with benign tumors, prostrate glands full of heavy metals and tissue with concentrations of chemicals are examples of fertile tissues that support parasitic growth. Hulda Clark's theory is that in the presence of propyl alcohol the shell of the cyst form of the parasite, metacercaria, is dissolved not in the intestine where it is intended but internal organs.

As soon as there are adult flukes living in the liver a growth factor, called ortho-phospho-tyrosine appears. Ortho- phospho-tyrosine is one of over two dozen cancer markers present in cancerous tissue. Additionally, the enzyme that makes ortho-phospho-tyrosine can be inhibited by genisteine, and this is why there may be such a success in the prevention and treatment of cancers with this substance.

The presence of propyl alcohol in the body allows the development of the fluke outside of the intestine. It is possible that the various parasitic stages produce the ortho-phospho-tyrosine in order to help themselves divide or perhaps induce the body to make it. Now with the presence of this growth factor the cells of the body start to divide, and this is the beginning of cancer.

Clark's theory focuses on eliminating the parasite from the body. Once these creatures are eliminated then the ortho-phospho-tyrosine disappears and so does the cancer.

Getting rid of the flukes in your body There are three natural herbs that are required. The first one is cloves; this will kill the parasite eggs; the second and third are wormwood leaves, (Artemisia) and a tincture of black walnut hulls, which kill the adult and development stages of at least 100 parasites including the culprit intestinal fluke.

As a side note it is very important to guarantee that the herbs and spices that you are buying are of good quality, otherwise this program to eliminate the flukes and the cancer will not be effective. Each of the three substances is discussed below.

The first, black walnut tincture, must be the extract of the green shells of the black walnuts, not the extract of the shells after they have turned brown. Health food stores should have such a tincture. It can be ordered from: "Blessed Herbs" in Oakham, Massachusetts 1-800-489-4372. The quantity, about 1 ounce, should be sufficient for the cure. The cost is about $6.00 for a one-ounce bottle. The second substance is wormwood with the botanical name of Artemisia absynthium. This plant has been used for the removal of intestinal worms for many years. The leaves are a silvery gray color and quite bitter. Wormwood is available in a combination with other herbs. One source that I have found is, "Pacific Botanicals" and the phone number is 1-503-479-7777 and their fax number is 1-503-479-5271, or it may be ordered from "Blessed Herbs" in Oakham, Massachusetts 1-800-489-4372. The reason that its sale is limited and it is not sold as a single ingredient is due to its mild toxicity. Even though for centuries it was one of the major ingredients of aperitifs and herb wines. The quantity is two bottles of 80 Wormwood combination capsules each. These capsules contain wormwood, male fern, quassia, and black walnut leaves. The quantity of Wormwood is only about 1/4 that of the combination capsules. This is because there is only about 25% wormwood in the combination capsules.

The third necessary ingredient is cloves. This is the common spice that is used in baking. It will need to be ground up in order to release its parasite killing properties. Buy whole cloves unground, as store bought "ground cloves" do not work. Their parasite killing properties evaporate very quickly. They can be ground with an inexpensive coffee grinder, About 100 capsules of cloves size 00 (double zero) are needed. Empty capsules are also available in most health food stores.

In review, you now have:
- One 30 cc bottle of pale green Black Walnut Hull Tincture
- 2 bottles of 80 Wormwood Combination capsules or 1/2 cup of Artemisia leaves.
- One bottle of 100 capsules of freshly ground cloves equals approximately 1/3 of a cup.Hulda Clark states in her book that there are no side effects when these herbs are taken in the prescribed doses and also there is no interference with other medication.

The dose of each of the herbs is as listed:

1. Black walnut tincture: Put in a beverage like water, milk, juice and take before meals on an empty stomach. The recommended dosage is as follows:

Day	Dosage Frequency
Day one	one (1) drop 4 times daily
Day two	two (2) drops 4 times daily
Day three	three (3) drops 4 times daily
Day four	four (4) drops 4 times daily
Day five	five (5) drops 4 times daily

Continue increasing until you reach 20 drops four times daily as shown below:

Day 20	twenty (20) drops 4 times daily
Days 20 to 90	twenty (20) drops 1 time daily

Maintenance: thirty (30) drops 2 times weekly for the rest of your life in case of re-infection.

2. Wormwood Combination capsules: take capsules before a meal with water.

Day	Dosage Frequency
Day one	one (1) capsule at nights before supper, 1 time daily
Day two	two (2) capsules at nights before supper, 1 time daily
Day three	three (3) capsules at nights before supper, 1 time daily

Continuing increasing in this manner until the 14th day as shown below:

Day fourteen	fourteen (14) capsules at nights before supper, 1 time daily
Day fifteen	fourteen (14) capsules at nights before supper, 1 time daily
Day sixteen	fourteen (14) capsules at nights before supper, 1 time daily

Maintenance: 14 capsules 2 times a week for the rest of your life in case of re-infection.

3. Cloves: Take as follows:

Day	Dosage Frequency
Day one	one (1) capsule 3 times daily
Day two	two (2) capsules 3 times daily
Day three	three (3) capsules 3 times daily
Day four	three (3) capsules 3 times daily
Day five	three (3) capsules 3 times daily
Day six	three (3) capsules 3 times daily
Day seven	three (3) capsules 3 times daily
Day eight	three (3) capsules 3 times daily

Day nine — three (3) capsules 3 times daily

Days ten to ninety — three (3) capsules 1 time daily

Maintenance: three 3 capsules 2 X a week for the rest of your life in case of re-infection.

The discoverer of this parasite elimination program, Hulda Clark, states that by the sixth day the intestinal flukes will be dead and the balance of the program (3 months) eliminates a variety of other parasites. It is crucial not to interrupt or quit this program before the sixth day. It is the intestinal fluke that apparently is responsible for the production of ortho-phospho-tyrosine, and cancer.

For more on this subject you can purchase Hulda Clark's book *The Cure for all Cancers*. This book is published by "ProMotion Publishing" 1-800-231-1776 and has a Library of Congress Card Catalog number RC268.C961098765. The cost of this book is approximately $20.00.

Inadequate Testing Procedures According to the well-respected internist, Dr. Leo Galland, conventional testing methods for parasite detection are often inadequate. Most tests look for parasites in the stool but overlook parasites living in the intestinal mucosa. As a result patients are given a false sense of security when they are told they do not have parasites. Scully and others report that a negative stool sample is not conclusive at ruling out parasites as the cause of illness. Clinical results have shown "diagnostic yield on up to three such stool examinations is usually no greater than 50%.

Biochemical Imbalances Parasitic symptoms are quite diverse as the body's biochemistry is thrown out of balance. Parasites consume many of the same nutrients needed by the patient. Vitamin B12 and folic acid deficiencies often result, while the parasite overburdens the liver by dumping ammonia into the blood stream. Ammonia will cause faulty signaling of the pituitary gland resulting in brain fog, confusion, headaches or hormonal imbalances that can affect the entire body.

Immune Suppression Parasites affect the patient's immune system by decreasing the production of secretory IgA antibodies, which represents the body's first line of defense. By activating an immune response, parasites overwork the immune system by increasing specific antibody reactions. This often leads to weakness and exhaustion of the immune system.

Parasites in Families Parasitic infections are often transmitted among family members. For this reason, it is extremely important to test the entire family for parasites and to treat each infected member to prevent relapse.

SECTION 1 REFERENCES

References for Lead

[1] Smith, M. A., Grant, L. D. & Sors, A. (1989). Lead exposure and child development: an international assessment. Kleeven Academic Publishers

[2] Silbergeld, E. K. (1992). Neurological perspective on lead toxicity. In Human Lead Exposure, ed H. L. Needleman, CRC Press

[3] National Research Council (US). (1993). Measuring lead exposure in infants children and other sensitive populations. National Academy Press, Washington DC

[4] Chemwatch Database. (1996) Lead Arsenate

[5] Alperstein, G., Reznik, R. & Duggin, G. (1991). Lead: Subtle forms and new modes of poisoning. The Medical Journal of Australia Vol 155 Sept 16.

[6] Berry, M., Garrard, J. & Greene, D. (1994). Reducing Lead Exposure in Australia. Commonwealth Department of Human Services and Health, Canberra

[7] Clark, H. R. (1995). The cure for all diseases. Pro Motion Publishing, San Diego California

[8] Needleman, H. L., Riess, J. A., Tobin, M., Biesecker, G. & Greenhouse, J.B. (1996). Bone Lead Levels and Delinquent Behavior. vol 275 No 5 JAMA. February 7. pgs. 363-369

[9] Gil, F. (1996). The science of the total environment.

[10] Fox, D. A. (1992). Visual and Auditory System Alterations following Developmental or Adult Lead. Exposure: a critical review. In Human Lead Exposure, ed H. L. Needleman, CRC Press

[11] Goldstein, G. W. (1992). Developmental neurobiology of lead toxicity. In Human Lead Exposure, ed H. L. Needleman, CRC Press

[12] Rice, D. C., (1992). Behavioural Impairment produced by developmental lead exposure: Evidence from primate research. In Human Lead Exposure, ed H. L. Needleman, CRC Press

[13] Matte, T. D., Landrigan P. J. & Baker E. L. (1992). Occupational Lead Exposure. In Human Lead Exposure, ed H. L. Needleman, CRC Press

[14] Wedeen R. P. (1992). Lead, the kidneys and hypertension. In Human Lead Exposure, ed H. L. Needleman, CRC Press

[15] Bellinger, D. & Needleman, H. L. (1992). Neurodevelopmental effects of low-level lead exposure in children. In Human Lead Exposure, ed H. L. Needleman, CRC Press

[16] Burchfile, J. L., Duffy, F. H., Bartels P. H., & Needleman, H. L. (1992). Low-level lead exposure: Effect on quantitative electroencephalography and correlation with neuropsychologic measures. In Human Lead Exposure, ed H. L. Needleman, CRC Press

[17] Schwartz, J. (1992). "Lead, blood pressure and cardio-vascular disease" In Human Lead Exposure, ed H. L. Needleman, CRC Press

[18] Schwartz, J. (1992). Low level health effects of lead: Growth, developmental and neurological disturbances. In Human Lead Exposure, ed H. L. Needleman, CRC Press

[19] Rutter, M. & Jones, R. (ed) Lead versus health: Sources and effects of low level lead exposure. Wiley medical Publications

[20] National Academy of Sciences. (1980). Lead in the Human Environment. Washington DC

[21] Castellino, N., Castellino, P. & Sannolo, N. (ed). (1995). Inorganic lead exposure. Lewis Publishers

[22] Hu, H., Pepper, L. & Goldman, R. (1991). Effects of repeated occupational exposure to lead. American Journal of Industrial Medicine V 20 pgs. 723-735

[23] Kim, R., Rotnitzky, A., Sparrow, D., Weiss, S. T., Wager, C. & Hu, H. (1996). Low level lead exposure and impairment of renal function. JAMA Vol 275 No 15 April. pg. 1177

[24] Fischbein, A. (1992). Occupational and environmental lead exposure. In Environmental and Occupational Medicine, 2nd edn. Ed W.N. Rom. Little, Brown & Co.

[25] Renpel, D. (1989). California occupational health program JAMA Vol 262 No 4.

[26] Repko, J. (1976). Behavioral toxicology of inorganic Lead. In Health Effects of Occupational Lead and Arsenic

Exposure — a symposium, ed.B. W. Carnow, US Dept of Health, Education and Welfare Public Health Service Divn of Surveillance Hazard Evaluation and Field Studies.

[27] Fanning, D. (1988). A mortality study of lead workers 1926 — 1985. In Archives of Environmental Health, Vol 43 No 3 May/June. pgs. 247-251.

[28] Barnett, M. (1982). A mortality study of lead workers 1925 — 76. In British Journal of Industrial Medicine Vol 39. pgs. 404-410

[29] Davies, J. M. (1984). Long-term mortality study of chromate pigment workers who suffered lead poisoning. In British Journal of Industrial Medicine, Vol 41. pgs. 170-178

[30] McMichael, A. J. & Johnson, H. M. (1982). Long term mortality profile of heavily exposed lead smelter workers. In Journal of Occupational Health, Vol 24 No 5.

[31] Winder, C. (1989). Reproductive and chromosomal effects of occupational exposure to lead in the male. In Reproductive Toxicology Review. Vol 7. pgs. 221-233.

[32] Schwartz, J. & Otto, D. (1987). Blood lead, hearing thresholds, and neurobehavioral development in children and youth. In Archives of Environmental Health Vol 42, No. 21 pgs 153-160, 1st May 1987.

[33] Fergusson, D. M., Hurwood, L. J. & Lynskey, M. T. (1997). Early dentine lead levels and educational outcomes at 18 years. In Journal of Child Psychology and Psychiatry, Vol 38 No 4. pgs. 471-478.

[34] NSW Workcover Authority. Occupational Medicine Handbook Ch 5 "Lead" pg. 58

[35] Royce, S. E. (1992). Lead toxicity. US Dept of Health and Human Services Agency for Toxic Substances and Disease Registry.

[36] Gatsonis, C. A.. & Needleman, H. L. (1992). Recent epidemiological studies of low-level lead exposure and the IQ of children: a meta-analytic review In Human Lead Exposure, ed H. L. Needleman, CRC Press

[37] Day, M. (1998) Lead in the womb. New Scientist Magazine. 23 May 1998 pg.7

[38] Werbach, M. F. (1997). Foundations of nutritional medicine. Third Line press, Tarzana California.

[39] Agency for Toxic Substances Disease Registrar. (1989). Toxicological profile of lead. US ATSDR.

[40] Salome, F. & Gulson, B. (1996). Lead paint management. Grad School of the Environment, Macquarie University

[41] Lanphear, Bruce P; Dietrich, Kim; Auinger, Peggy; Cox, Christopher. (2000) Cognitive Deficits Associated with Blood Lead Concentrations <10 µg/dL in US Children and Adolescents, Public Health Reports Nov 2000, Volume 115, 521-529; phr.oupjournals.org/cgi/reprint/115/6/521.pdf

[42] Walsh, William J; Usman, Anju; Tarpey, Jeffrey; and Kelly, Tanika. (2001) Metallothionein And AutismPfeiffer Treatment Center, Health Research Institute, Naperville, Illinois USA. The booklet can be ordered from info@HRIPTC.org or via the website *www.hriptc.org* for US$20 + postage but is not web-published. October 2001

[43] Wentzel, Michael, Democrat & Chronicle, 25/2/02, UR (University of Rochester) links childhood lead to osteoporosis *www.democratandchronicle.com/news/0225story2_news.shtml*

References for Chlorinated Water

[1] Fackelmann, K.A., Hints of a chlorine-cancer connection. Science News, July 11, 1992;142:23.

[2] Flaten, Trond Peter. Chlorination of drinking water and cancer incidence in Norway. International Journal of Epidemiology, 1992;21(1):6-15.

[3] Messina, Virginia. Chlorine and cancer. Good Medicine, Winter 1994;8-9.

[4] Morris, Robert D. Chlorination, Chlorination by-products and cancer. American Journal of Public Health, July 1992;82(7):955-963.

[5] Rothery, S.P., et al. Hazards of chlorine to asthmatic patients. British Journal of General Practice, Jan, 1991;39.

[6] Shaw, Gary M., et al. Chlorinated water exposures and congenital cardiac anomalies. Epidemiology, November 1991;2(6):459-460.

References for Root Canal

[1] Root Canals — The Inside Story, by Hal A. Huggins, DDS, MS.

[2] Uninformed Consent, by Hal A. Huggins, DDS, MS and Thomas Levy, M.D., J.D., 1998.

[3] Cancer: A Second Opinion, by Josef M. Issels, M.D., 1999 Avery Publishing Group, N.Y.

"All truth passes through three stages. First, it is ridiculed. Second it is violently opposed. Third, it is accepted as being self-evident."

Arthur Schopenhauer (1788-1860)

Section 2

DESTROYING CANCER

Destroying the cancer is certainly a major priority in any proposed cancer program. However, various considerations come into play, which will influence selecting the best methods for addressing your particular issues. Like anything else in life every thing has its limitations and conventional and alternative medicines are no exception. The following information is presented to make cancer patients aware of innovative technologies both old and new that have proven effective. The more treatment options available the better the odds of reversing the disease process. Although extremely vital, these options represent just one part of the big puzzle.

This cancer ultimately developed because of a breakdown of the immune system. Even if the cancer was totally eradicated there still remains the un-nerving fact that the same factors that caused the cancer are still present! The environment of the body *must* be dealt with to achieve a long lasting successful outcome. In most cases, those patients who choose the traditional path of surgery, chemotherapy and radiation without addressing the issues that set the stage for causing the cancer are living with a false sense of security.

To assist patients in establishing a treatment protocol, an asterisk appears after each technique and supplement used in reversing the stage III ovarian cancer. Regardless of what type of cancer a patient has the noted approach can be applied. To maximize effectiveness each substance used must be tested.

RIFE GENERATOR*

Raymond Royal Rife was a brilliant researcher who invented a high-powered microscope in 1929, which enabled him to view cancer viruses and other pathogens. His microscope was unique in that it stained the pathogens with light. A prism rotated very slowly until the pathogen absorbed the specific color of light at which the organism vibrated. Doctor Rife painstakingly determined the vibratory rates of fifty-two different disease-causing organisms. One of Rife's major discoveries was the cancer causing virus' mortal oscillatory frequency. Doctor Rife observed that when the color or frequency of light that illuminated the cancer virus matched exactly its vibratory frequency the cancer virus exploded. This find enabled him to work with Lee De Forest, the inventor of the vacuum tube, to construct a generating device that could produce and broadcast the specific frequencies. The Rife Generator was consistently able to successfully treat cancer as well as many other common diseases. The mortal frequency had the distinct advantage of destroying the pathogen without the microorganism developing any resistance, which often occurred with the use of drugs. Rife's greatest achievement came in 1934. Under the auspices of the University of Southern California, Dr. Rife and a group of distinguished scientists were given sixteen terminally ill cancer patients. In 130 days all sixteen-cancer patients were cured. It is difficult to believe that this historic breakthrough in medicine quickly brought the wrath of the FDA, pharmaceutical companies and AMA to bring an end to such treatment. It was astutely concluded by powerful interests that Rife's discovery would destroy the pharmaceutical Industry, as it existed in the 1930's.

Today, many Rife type devices or function generators are available for purchase. However, not all are accurate. A word of caution before purchasing such a device: make sure that the unit has been used successfully on many different medical maladies. I have personally used the Rife technology (function generators are available from ICNR, Inc. 1-800-272-2323) successfully since 1997. This was the year my wife had breast cancer. The first surgical procedure involved a lumpectomy. The pathology report stated that the surgeon missed a margin, that is, there were cancer cells remaining in the area of the incision. Two months later a second surgery removed the remaining cancerous tissue. During the two-month period between surgeries my wife used the Rife machine twice a day. The second pathology report stated that there were no cancer cells in the area.

On December 9, 2002, my wife was diagnosed with stage III ovarian cancer when she had surgery for what we were led to believe were fibroid tumors. The good news is that I was able to reverse the remaining cancer cells in just two months with alternative therapies (Rife- I brought the unit into the hospital and treated my wife immediately after surgery; organic coffee enemas-caffeinated of course-hold the cream and sugar; metabolic typing diet; detox herbs, supplements galore). Her cancer antigen tumor marker, CA 125, was 840 (normal 0-20) before surgery. It dropped to 130 two weeks after surgery and is now 2.2. Her LASA-P

(Lipid Associated Sialic Acid in Plasma), which is another tumor marker, was 17.2 down from 24 (normal high is 23). Both tests are available from Dianon: 200 Watson Boulevard, Stratford, CT 06615, Phone: 1-800-328-2666, 1-203-381-4000, Fax: 1-203-381-4079. Your doctor can register by calling and providing the necessary information.

We then sought out IPT (Insulin Potentiation Therapy), ozone, hydrogen peroxide, irradiation of blood with ultraviolet and infrared spectrum light, intravenous vitamin C and photo activated substances, which are given intravenously to impregnate the cancer cells with natural and synthetic substances. These substances when exposed to photonic energy cause a superoxidation to occur within the cancer cells. This process disrupts the metabolism of the cancer cells resulting in the cell's death without harming the normal cells.

To assist in diagnosing the presence and location of the remaining cancer cells, I had the surgeon get me a piece of the tumor. Then I had the frequency of the tumor imprinted into a vial of distilled water. Since waster is a crystal, it will store the frequency. Imprinting can be accomplished by means of a Vega, Dermatron, Interro or similar unit. By means of Direct Resonance Testing, I used this vial to locate exactly where the metastasis was and to determine what substances will work. Treatment went smoothly and there were no adverse reactions to the multiple techniques. Since an extensive detoxification program was completed prior to the IPT treatments, my wife's body was able to handle the toxins liberated from the treatment. Other than feeling a little tired from sitting during the three-hour sessions, my wife felt a sense of well-being and the nurses could not believe that her blood did not look like a typical cancer patient's — viscous and deep red.

INSULIN POTENTIATION THERAPY (IPT)*

A Mexican physician developed IPT treatment in the early 1900's. The underlying concept was to gain rapid access to the intracellular metabolism of pathogens such as viruses, bacteria, funguses and cancer cells. This therapy has been successful in the treatment of viruses like polio, cancer and many other difficult diseases. IPT use is particularly effective in the treatment of cancer because cancer cells have been shown to have ten times more insulin receptors plus insulin-like growth-factor receptors than normal cells. The benefit of insulin is that it makes all cells, cancer, viruses, bacteria, and fungi vulnerable to intracellular penetration. In addition, insulin modifies the growth characteristics in cancer cells by stimulating less active cancer cells into the growth phase thus making them more vulnerable to anticancer agents.

By intravenous administration of insulin, the fasting blood sugar levels are lowered to a working therapeutic window (10 to 12 minutes). This window is an individualized hypoglycemic event (observable signs and symptoms: chills, sweating, pale complexion, weakness, dizziness, jitteriness, and mild headache) in each patient. During transition into this hypoglycemic state, the patient's vital blood sugar levels and blood pressure signs are carefully monitored.

During the hypoglycemic event, proprietary photo activated substances, which are selective for cancer, are intravenously infused. The patient is then given glucose in the form of Gatorade® to elevate their blood sugar. With the restoration of the blood sugar, the signs and symptoms disappear. Quinoxide is then infused intravenously over a 15-minute period to create a highly oxidative environment, which favors an oxidative assault on cancer cells. Following the Quinoxide infusion, 250 to 300 cc of the patient's blood is withdrawn via the intravenous line and treated with ozone (minor auto-hemotherapy) and then passed through a specialized photon pump, which generates an infrared to ultraviolet spectrum of light. This process activates the photosensitive substances in all cells but primarily in cancer cells. A cascade response of the anti-oxidative system is set in motion. This anti-oxidative system is intact in all healthy cells as a self-protective mechanism. Cancer cells lack this protective mechanism and self-destruct (Apoptosis). Depending on the health of the patient, IPT treatment can be given once or three times a week. The most frequent side effects experienced by patients are chills and fever which are acceptable and denote a favorable response. In my personal experience the IPT treatment works much more effectively when the body is detoxified prior, during and after treatment. By removing excess toxins, the immune system (liver, kidneys, white blood cells, spleen, thymus gland and thyroid gland) can more easily remove the waste products generated by the IPT treatment. The detoxification process will reduce or even eliminate the adverse side effects.

OXIDATIVE THERAPY*

Most biochemical reactions in the body are balanced through redox mechanisms. Redox means (red)uction (ox)idation. Anytime a substance is reduced (chemically changed) something else must be oxidized (chemically changed the other way for the reactions to stay in balance. As an example, oxidation is the process that causes rust (slow oxidation) or fire (rapid oxidation). In the body some types of oxidation are thought to be harmful because they produce free radicals. We know there can be no life if oxidation does not occur. Oxidation is the process through which the body converts sugar into energy. The body also uses oxidation as the first line of defense against bacteria, viruses, yeast and parasites. Even breathing oxygen is an oxidative process. Without oxygen for more that six minutes irreversible brain cell damage will result. When we use the principle of oxidation to bring about improvement in the body it is referred to as Oxidative Therapy. Hydrogen peroxide also helps regulate certain chemicals necessary to operate the brain and nervous system. It is also used in the defense system of the body to kill bacteria, viruses, yeast and parasites. It plays an important role in regulating the immune system.

Oxidative Therapy is administered by the intravenous infusion of a pure diluted mixture of hydrogen peroxide (.0375% or lower) and dextrose (sugar) solution. Doses of between 50 to 500ml are infused into a large vein, usually in the arm, over a period of one to three hours. The therapy is an effective approach when used on alternate days between Insulin Potentiation Therapy. It can also be effective on a daily basis with acute illnesses like pneumonia or the flu. Oxidative therapy is safe when administered properly.

A number of substances are known to cause oxidation in the body, however, the most important of these is hydrogen peroxide (H_2O_2). Although a natural substance made in the body, it is still considered a drug when used in Oxidative Therapy. Hydrogen Peroxide, when exposed to blood or other body fluids containing the enzyme catalyase, causes it to split into oxygen and water. The foaming action that occurs when hydrogen peroxide is applied to a wound is the result of the action of catalyase acting on the hydrogen peroxide to release the oxygen. A small amount of hydrogen peroxide can supply a large quantity of oxygen to the tissues.

Injections of hydrogen peroxide are not new in medicine. In 1920, Dr. T.H. Oliver reported intravenous use of hydrogen peroxide in the respected British medical journal, Lancet. Patients with influenza and pneumonia were treated with hydrogen peroxide infusions with very good results. The use of hydrogen peroxide injections to generate oxygen in the body has been studied and reported by physicians at major medical research centers, universities (Baylor, Yale, Harvard, UCLA,) in the United States and throughout the world (England, Japan, Germany, Sweden, Russia, Canada, and Nova Scotia). Today, between 50 and 100 scientific articles are published each month about the chemical and biological effects of hydrogen peroxide. In more recent times, Charles H. Farr, Ph.D., at an International Medical Symposium in Czechoslovakia, reported the "Therapeutic Use of Hydrogen Peroxide." The increased worldwide use of hydrogen peroxide was reflected in the fact that representatives attended the conference from 26 different countries.

Hydrogen peroxide is produced in the body in different amounts for different purposes. It is part of a system that uses oxygen for breathing. It is part of a system that helps the body regulate all living cell membranes. It functions as a hormonal regulator to produce several hormonal substances such as: estrogen, progesterone, and thyroid. It is important in the regulation of blood sugar and the production of energy in all cells.

PHOTODYNAMIC THERAPY*

Photodynamic therapy uses light to fight cancer. Of course, light by itself cannot kill cancer cells. However, if patients are pre-treated with a sensitizer drug and are then administered light of a certain wavelength, their cancer cells will die by the millions. This is because the energy of the beam of light activates the sensitizer substance within the cancer cell. The reaction causes the release of singlet oxygen, a kind of free radical. This process does not harm normal cells for two reasons: first healthy cells have their antioxidant mechanism intact and can deal with the singlet oxygen. Second, the sensitizing drug accumulates only in cancer and other abnormal tissues, which do not have an adequate antioxidant system to neutralize the free radical oxygen.

This innovative approach focuses on destroying the cancer without damaging the normal cells. The sensitizing agents presently used are third generation and eliminate the previous shortcomings. The new agents are derived from green plants (algae), which makes them a much more sensitive, effective and less toxic substance.

THE RATIONAL FOR TAKING SO MANY SUPPLEMENTS

The process of degeneration is at its maximum level in the cancer patient! The fact that cancer is present is a verification of poor overall health. The proposed program helps the body *regenerate* by placing high quality fuel (unprocessed food and natural supplements) into the system. A rule of thumb is that the sicker the patient the longer the healing time and the more supplements will be required, and strict adherence to dietary recommendations will be absolutely essential. In most cases these changes represent a 180-degree change from the patient's past dietary habits.

This author's experience confirms that *testing each supplement's biocompatibility speeds up the healing process*, reduces the number of pills required and saves time and money. Using the same protocol with every patient is not realistic. In the 1930's Roger Williams, a Ph.D., from the University of Texas, discovered that every person is a chemical individual. With today's technology, it is not necessary to take a shotgun approach with supplements. Sensitive computerized equipment can quickly measure a supplement's compatibility with the patient's energy field. Applied Kinesiology, Autonomic Response Testing and cranial rhythm can also be used to determine biocompatibility. Clinically, I have found that cranial rhythm analysis is the most accurate. The following description guides the user through the required steps.

TESTING PROCEDURES TO PROPERLY DETERMINE BIOCOMPATIBILITY OF SUBSTANCES

Unfortunately even alternative practitioners prescribe various therapies and nutritional supplements because some researcher statistically found that a particular selection of supplements or technique worked well for a percentage of people regarding a particular form of cancer. I have been practicing alternative and complementary health care since 1969 and come to realize that every patient is a chemical individual and *must* be treated as such. Even though a particular substance or technique shows statistical success, it does not necessarily mean that it will work for you.

The paradigm that will be presented is based on actual clinical successes. The methodology focuses on the concept of balancing energy patterns of each patient. Methods are presently available in the form of computerized systems (Biotron, BodyScan, Interro, Vega) that enable testing of acupuncture meridians and balancing energy deficiencies with nutritional supplements. Substances can also be quickly tested by means of assessing the amplitude of the cranial rhythm after the substance is placed on the patient. Every person has an energy field or aura, which is an extension of his or her autonomic nervous system (peripheral nervous system). It is easy for anyone trained in palpating the cranial motion (or locate someone who is trained) to employ the technique. This skull motion is present in everyone. It represents the pumping mechanism to move cerebrospinal fluid around the head and down the spinal cord. Once the practitioner feels the amplitude of the skull, he or she has established a baseline against which all comparisons are made. Utilizing this technique will help reduce many variable factors that may influence test results obtained by using muscle testing (Applied Kinesiology, Autonomic Response Testing) and other methods.

SMITH CRANIAL MOTION ANALYSIS (SCMA)*

The procedure is performed by the following steps:

Have the patient lie comfortably in a supine position with their neck supported by a small cushion or rolled towel. The palm of each hand is gently placed on each side of the patient's head approximating the greater lateral convexity. The palms barely touch the hair or if bald *very lightly* on the skin. The objective is to perceive the gentle lateral expansion and contraction of the skull. Care is taken to perceive the symmetry of the motion: large bilateral robust amplitude; bilaterally weak amplitude; unilateral weakness; unilateral robust motion; diagonal motion or very little motion. If motion is almost non-perceptible or if the motion feels chaotic (like holding a bag of live worms), the individual needs a cranial adjustment prior to conducting the test. Most individuals will exhibit good motion and permit testing. By allowing the pumping mechanism to complete several cycles, a baseline motion is established.

After the baseline rhythm is established, each supplement is placed on the chest one at a time and the amplitude is reassessed. If the motion *distorts* the baseline motion felt, then that particular supplement will *not* benefit the patient's healing process. Only those supplements that support the basic skull motion's symmetry will be in synchronization with the patient's healing mechanism.

After each supplement is tested, the practitioner can determine the exact dosage of each supplement and when it should be taken. While the specific supplement is still on the patient, the practitioner silently asks him or herself various dosage schedules: for example; one capsule three times a day; two capsules three times per day, etc. The dosage that distorts the cranial rhythm is not used but the one before is. Retest in your mind to clarify the correctness by repeating the previous dosage and assessing if the cranial rhythm still remains balanced. If perception becomes clouded, temporarily remove hands, rub palms together and reposition.

The same procedure can be used to determine when to take the nutrients. Just silently ask with meals and assess the cranial rhythm. Then silently ask between meals. One can do the same for upon arising, between breakfast and lunch, between lunch and dinner and before bedtime.

Once all supplements have been tested individually, then all those which tested positive must be tested together to determine if they will *all* work synergistically. If when all tested, there is a distortion, then retest by removing one supplement at a time from the patient to determine if all the remaining ones will work together. This may take a little time since various combinations must be tested. The correct combination will maintain a symmetrical motion.

- Supplements that test good alone but do not test positive with the others must be given separately. As the patient heals, periodic retesting must be performed to assess dosages and combinations. During the first three months, testing should be performed every two to three weeks. Nutrient compatibility and combinations will change during reassessment sessions.

This SCMA (Smith Cranial Motion Analysis) will be greatly enhanced when followed up with Dr. Yoshiaki Omura's Selective Drug Enhancement Uptake Method. Omura has clinically mapped out the accurate organ representation areas on each palm surface that correspond to particular organs and regions of the body. By stimulating the specific organ representation areas on the hands for ten minutes (prolonged stimulation achieves better results) following ingestion of effective medications and/or nutrients, the substance(s) will concentrate in the pathological part of the body while reducing drug uptake to the normal body parts. To facilitate diagnosis of the underlying causes of cancer and other degenerative diseases, Dr. Omura developed the Bi-Digital O-Ring Test. Omura is credited as the originator of the two-minute, non-invasive screening test for cancer using laser beam technology. His test often detects early stages of various cancers even when standard medical tests fail. Dr. Omura offers regular seminars to teach his advanced Bi-Digital O-Ring Testing and Selective Drug Uptake Enhancement Method to professionals (contact information: 1-212-781-6262). Combining the two techniques results in the most effective approach to target healing ever achieved in medicine. Omura's acupuncture hand chart is available from M.I.C. International Corp. 1-201-432-1717.

The end result will be a custom nutritional program that will work exceptionally fast. By properly selecting a program one will save countless amounts of money by avoiding shotgun nutritional programs with the hope that they will work. This approach can be used for medications, antioxidants, herbs, enzymes, homeopathic remedies, foods, natural or synthetic substances to be used with Insulin Potentiation Therapy and even dental materials to be placed in the teeth. In reality, the closer one comes to the truth the more simplistic the solution. It is amazing how accurate this process is.

The following supplements are recommended to take the burden off of the pancreas, liver and kidneys and provide essential enzymes to allow the body to function more efficiently. The supplements help the immune system to more effectively destroy the cancer, re-establish mineral and pH (acid/base) balance and enhance calcium metabolism. These processes depend on a daily supply of high quality nutrients and food.

Agaricus Blazei Murill (ABM) Mushroom In the 1970's researchers noticed that an unusual percentage of people in a small town in Brazil (Piedate, in Sao Paulo) had few serious diseases related to aging. The common denominator among these people was their consumption of the ABM (Agaricus Blazei Murill) mushroom known to the locals as 'Cogumelo de Deus' or 'Mushroom of God'.

Researchers have isolated large amounts of polysaccharides (multiple molecules of simple sugar molecules chained together to form more complex sugars) in this mushroom, which appear to significantly boost the immune system. The polysaccharides have been shown to activate the immune system in several ways. First, they stimulate white blood cells known as macrophages, which destroy viruses, bacteria, and perhaps even cancer cells, by engulfing and digesting them and second, by stimulating lymphocyte T-cell and Helper T-cell production.

The polysaccharide contained in the ABM mushroom also stimulates production of interferon and interleukin that indirectly function to destroy and prevent the proliferation of cancer cells. Additionally, ABM is also a powerful antiviral agent that prevents viruses from entering tissues. Other mushrooms like Shiitake, Maitake and Reishi also contain these polysaccharides.

ABM is also known as Himematsutake and can be used in cooking the same way as other mushrooms. Daily dosage for normal body maintenance and prevention is about 6 grams (about 1/4 of a dry mushroom) or 40 grams (approx. 2 mushrooms) for serious illnesses. Tea is also a popular way of taking the mushroom. Use about one (1) mushroom per liter (1 quart) and boil it for an hour. Drink one cup a day, warm or cold. Take a natural form of vitamin C (Cataplex C derived from green buckwheat or Foodform® C — both available from ICNR, Inc. 1-800-272-2323) in conjunction with medicinal mushrooms to assist in the absorption of the beneficial properties of the mushroom.

Normally, the polysaccharides found in fungus only affect solid cancers, however the polysaccharide in ABM is effective against Ehrich's ascites carcinoma, sigmoid colon cancer, ovarian cancer, breast cancer, lung cancer, and liver cancer as well as solid cancers.

In Japan, ABM was found to eliminate all cancerous tumors in 90% of experimental mice. Additionally, when the mice were fed ABM as a preventative and then injected with a very powerful cancer-causing agent (Sarcoma 180), 99.4% of them showed no tumor growth. Conventional medicine has nothing as powerful as this.

The studies in Japan showed ABM to be 80% more effective than the world's number one cancer drug, PSK. It contains much higher levels of beta glucans than the other medicinal mushrooms (Maitake, Shiitake, and Reishi). It stimulates NK (Natural Killer) cell activity at a rate higher than MGN-3.

The studies in Japan were so successful that today Japan is now importing over 90% of the available ABM from Brazil.

The ABM mushroom is available in the US. Check out the following links: ABM freeze dried extract in capsules: *www.hplus.com/a36.html To order mushrooms in bulk, wholesale from China: www.abmcn.com/.* Jana Shiloh, a homeopathic consultant in Arizona handles all manner of Agaricus products. Write to *life@sedona.net* or visit her web site: *www.alternative-health-4u.com* or phone her at 1-888-282-9362. One of the largest suppliers in the world is *www.agaricus.net.*

Enzyme Therapy* Pancreatic enzymes dissolve the outer protein covering that enables cancer cells to avoid attack by the immune system. The pancreas is a vital organ in the prevention of cancer. In the 1960's William Donald Kelly, a dentist from Texas, had pancreatic cancer and was given a death sentence by the medical establishment. He discovered that the placenta grows like cancer cells to rapidly attach the developing fetus to the uterine wall. This process abruptly stops by the seventh week. Also of interest, the pancreas in the developing fetus starts working at exactly the seventh week. Dr. Kelly theorized that the presence of the pancreatic enzymes was responsible for turning off the "cancerous" growth of the placenta. An interesting footnote, diabetics get cancer more often than people with normal, functioning pancreases.

It is theorized that with solid tumors, enzyme therapy slowly works to degrade the outer cell walls of cancer cells, reducing growth and making other treatments more effective. By dissolving the protective protein covering, the immune system can now recognize the exposed tumor cells and destroy them.

In Leukemia studies (Cancer Research, vol. 32, pp. 280-284, 1972) three out of five patients responded to enzymatic therapy in conjunction with their anti-leukemic drugs and went into remission. They also report that one patient with AML achieved remission by enzyme therapy alone. The enzyme *A. oryzae* appeared to activate auto-cytotoxicity, an immune response that selectively destroys cancerous cells.

We recommend the use of the product by Advanced Formula, ProactEnz (each capsule contains 607mg of physioProtease- one bottle contains 60 vegetarian capsules — both available from *www.icnr.com*).

Garlic[*] More has been written about the wonderful benefits of garlic than any other food. Its history dates back 3,500 years: Hippocrates, the father of medicine, was the first to write that garlic was an excellent medicine for eliminating tumors. Recent studies on garlic have shown it to be:

- Insecticidal — kills insects.
- Parasiticidal — eliminates parasites.
- Antibacterial — a wide spectrum antibiotic that doesn't kill the good bacteria.
- Antifungal — eliminates fungal growth.
- Antitumor — eliminates various tumors
- Hypoglycemic — lowers sugar levels in the blood
- Hypolipidemic — lowers harmful fat levels in the blood
- Antiatherosclerotic — eliminates clogging of the arteries and plaque buildup, lowering cholesterol and triglyceride levels

Additionally, garlic, containing germanium, helps tissues hold more oxygen, but is much less toxic than the expensive forms of germanium prescribed by physicians.

According to Dr. David G. Williams in his publication, *Secrets of Life Extension: 10 Simple All-Natural Steps to Achieving Your Maximum Lifespan*, garlic extract was responsible for normalizing T-cell proportions, reducing diarrhea, fever, Candidiasis, and occurrences of genital herpes, and restoring natural killer (NK) cell activity. The report, by the way, was published only in Germany.

According to Dr. Schulze, he's had a number of colon cancers dry up and die simply through a thorough colon cleanse and large doses of garlic. Garlic comes to us in many forms, yet most of them found in health food stores contain mostly vegetable oil, very little garlic, and have been over-processed. The best brand name garlic supplements on the market are from MediHerb®, which is available either in tablet form (5000mg/tab – 60 tabs/bottle) or liquid form (200ml/bottle) derived from fresh garlic bulb in a 1:1 extract. *Both products are available from ICNR, Inc. Recommended serving 5ml or one teaspoonful mixed with juice once a day. Other Ingredients:* Purified water and 45% alcohol.

Caution: Contraindicated in lactation. Not to be used during pregnancy unless otherwise directed by a qualified health care practitioner. It has been discovered that the diallyl sulfide in garlic reduces the formation of nitrosamines (carcinogens) in the liver. (*Cancer Research,* 1988; 48:23)

Penn State researchers have discovered that the anti-tumor activity of garlic can be destroyed by one minute of microwaving to forty-five minutes of oven roasting. *Cooking kills garlic's anti-tumor properties.* However, the good news is it doesn't have to. For one thing, if you have cancer, avoid using your microwave entirely and do not even use it to heat water. Next, chop up your garlic and let it set for 10 minutes before adding it to anything about to be cooked. This enables naturally present enzymes in the garlic to start a chemical reaction producing the compounds that fight tumors. Even better still, chop it up, let it sit, and add it only before serving. There are cases on record where cancer was beaten with a good detoxification program and garlic alone. It's not just for Italians any more.

Ellagic Acid[*] This acid is found in red raspberries, strawberries, blue berries, and certain nuts. Research articles have appeared as early as 1967 on the effectiveness of this compound on various types of cancer. In 1999, the Hollings Cancer Institute at the University of South Carolina completed a study showing that ellagic acid:

- Stops cancer cells from dividing in 48 hours
- Causes normal cell death (apoptosis) within 72 hours in cases of breast, pancreas, esophageal, skin, colon and prostate cancers
- Prevents the destruction of the p53 gene that leads to cancer
- Caused apoptosis (normal cell death) in exposed HPV (human papilloma virus)
- One cup (150 grams) per day of red raspberries prevents the development of cancer cells.

From Dr. Glen Halvorson's Book, *Chemopreventive Properties of Phytochemicals*, we learn that ellagic acid:

- is anti-bacterial and destroys the H. pylori bacteria responsible for stomach ulcers
- protects the liver and liver function
- binds with carcinogens (chemicals that cause cancer) making them inactive
- prevents carcinogens from binding to DNA
- reduces glucose levels, aids in management of diabetes

Raspberries contain the highest amounts of ellagic acid, and it doesn't matter if the fruit is boiled, baked, canned, sugared, dehydrated, or fresh, the ellagic acid is still potent.

One of the most amazing things about raspberries is that one-cup per week stops prostate cancers (all prostate cancers) from growing for one week. Currently at the Hollings Cancer Institute they are patenting a process that extracts the ellagic acid from raspberries and, hopefully, it will not be destroyed in the stomach (ellagic acid, so far, *cannot be taken as a supplement, and must be eaten as the fruit*) and they are conducting a double blind (neither patient nor physician knows who's taking what) study involving 500 cervical cancer patients. Please note: if you are eating raspberries for their ellagic acid you must eat them on an empty stomach, before you eat anything else, or eat them in yogurt, as the curdling of the yogurt in the stomach will protect them. If your fruit sits in your stomach too long, because you've eaten something prior, stomach acid will destroy its healthful properties. To read more about this wonderful food, go to: *www.red-raspberry.org/*. Whenever possible purchase organic berries.

Graviola* The following article appeared in a newsletter published by Health Sciences Institute. *Billion-dollar drug company nearly squashes astounding research on natural cancer killer; Colon and breast cancer conquered with miracle tree from the Amazon found to be 10,000 times stronger than chemotherapy*

Since our inception in 1996, Health Sciences Institute has scoured the world to find cutting-edge treatments few people have access to or have even heard about. And sometimes, what we uncover startles even the medical mavericks on our board.

Two months ago, we learned about an astounding cancer-fighting tree from the Amazon that has literally sent shock waves through the HSI network.

Today, the future of cancer treatment and the chances of survival look more promising than ever. There's a healing tree that grows deep within the Amazon rain forest in South America that could literally change how you, your doctor, and possibly the rest of the world think about curing cancer. With extracts from this powerful tree, it may now be possible to:

- conquer cancer safely and effectively with an all-natural therapy that doesn't cause extreme nausea, weight loss, and hair loss
- protect your immune system and evade deadly infections
- feel strong and healthy throughout the course of treatment
- boost your energy and improve your outlook on life

Through a series of confidential communications involving a researcher from one of America's largest pharmaceutical companies, this ancient tree's anti-cancerous properties have recently come to light. Although not yet tested in human trials, the tree has been studied in more than 20 laboratory tests since the 1970s, where it's been shown to:

- effectively target and kill malignant cells in 12 different types of cancer, including colon, breast, prostate, lung, and pancreatic cancer
- be 10,000 times stronger in killing colon cancer cells than Adriamycin, a commonly used chemotherapeutic drug
- selectively hunt down and kill cancer cells without harming healthy cells, unlike chemotherapy

So why isn't every health publication extolling the benefits of this treatment? Why hasn't it been made widely available throughout the natural-medicine community? And, if it's only half as promising as it appears to be, why isn't every oncologist at every major hospital insisting on using it on all his patients? Especially when you consider that since the early 1990s, extensive independent research — including research by one of today's leading drug companies and by the National Cancer Institute — confirms that the tree's chemical extracts attack and destroy cancer cells with lethal precision.

The answer to these difficult questions can only be explained by recounting a disturbing story we recently uncovered. More than anything else we've reported on this year, the story of this Amazon cancer treatment reinforces the need for groups like HSI and illustrates how easily our options for medical treatment are controlled by money and power.

News of this amazing tree was nearly lost forever A confidential source, whose account we've been able to independently confirm, revealed that a billion-dollar drug company in the United States tried for nearly seven years to synthesize two of the tree's most powerful anti-cancerous chemicals. In the early 1990s, behind lock and key, this well-known drug giant began searching for a cure for cancer — while preciously guarding their opportunity to patent it and, therefore, profit from it.

Research focused on a legendary healing tree called Graviola. Parts of the tree — including the bark, leaves, roots, fruit, and fruit seeds — had been used for centuries by medicine men and native Indians in South America to treat heart disease, asthma, liver problems, and arthritis. Going on little documented scientific evidence, the company poured money and resources into testing Graviola's anti-cancerous properties — and they were shocked by the results. Graviola was a cancer-killing dynamo. But that's where the story of Graviola nearly ended.

The pharmaceutical company had a big problem. They'd spent years trying to isolate and create man-made duplicates of two of the tree's most powerful chemicals. But they'd hit a brick wall. They couldn't replicate the original. And they couldn't sell the tree extract itself profitably — because federal law mandates that natural substances can't be patented. That meant the company couldn't protect its profits on the project it had poured millions of dollars and nearly seven years of research into. *As the dream of big profits evaporated, testing on Graviola came to a screeching halt.*

Gravizon* Graviola, Una de Gato, Pau d' Arco, Jatoba, Jurubeda, Sangre de Drago, Camu Camu, Dong Quai, Quebra Pedra, Alfalfa, Boldo, Artichocke, Soy, Safflower, Tangerine Peel, Aquilaria, Samambala, Sarsaparilla, Peach Kernel, Dalergia, Bitter Orange, Manaca, Tayuya, Catuaba, Suma, Iporuru, Abuta, Espinherira Santa, Muira Puama.
Caution: Not intended for use during pregnancy.
Available from: ICNR, Inc. 1-800-272-2323 or order directly *www.icnr.com*

Coral Calcium It is important to recognize that the Japanese and many people around the world use two broad, but distinct types of coral calcium as health giving supplements. The first type is fossilized calcium that has been deposited on the landmass, or washed up on to beaches. The second type is taken directly from the seabed. It is marine bed coral. This seabed coral is the coral that has dropped from the reef or is processed by reef inhabitants. This type of "coral sand" has been washed to the ocean floor by wave actions. Marine coral is closer in composition to the living forms of corals, because many minerals and organic elements are retained, in comparison to fossilized, land-based coral.

There are important differences in composition between fossilized (land-based) coral and marine (sea-bed) coral. Marine coral contains more magnesium, and the balance of calcium (24%) to magnesium (12%) content of this second type of marine coral is close to 2:1. This 2 to 1 ratio is the ideal ratio for calcium and magnesium intake in the human diet. Robert Barefoot's research has led him to believe strongly that the natural, magnesium enriched, marine coral is to be strongly preferred as a health giving supplement over land based (fossilized coral), which contains less than 1% magnesium. This superiority is due to its retained, ideal, ionic balance of calcium and magnesium in a 2:1 ratio, and the fact that a host of other nutrients were also washed out of fossilized coral during weathering processes.

Calcium Deficiency Syndrome In fact, over 200 degenerative diseases and medical conditions have been linked to calcium deficiency. Among them are:

- Alzheimer's Disease
- Angina
- Arteriosclerosis
- Arthritis
- Bone Spurs
- Cancer
- Chronic Fatigue Syndrome
- Diabetes
- Eczema
- Fibromyalgia
- Gallstones
- Gout
- Headaches
- Heart Disease
- Hiatal Hernia
- High Cholesterol
- Hypertension
- Joint Pain
- Kidney Stones
- Lupus
- Muscle Cramps
- Osteoporosis

Frequent hives, chronic fatigue, canker and cold sores, muscle cramps (Charlie Horses), and itchy skin may all be symptoms of calcium deficiency.

The primary cause of calcium deficiency is diet. The Standard American Diet (SAD) typically consists of high-fat, high-protein, high-phosphate, high sodium foods and beverages.

Examples include red meats, refined grains, heavily processed foods, bakery goods and soft drinks (especially cola drinks which contain large amounts of *phosphoric acid*). This is an over-acidic diet, and this upsets the body's acid/alkaline balance by draining our body of alkaline minerals, like calcium.

A number of substances in our food can inhibit the absorption of calcium:

- Phytic acid, found in bran, whole cereals and raw vegetables; phytic acid is destroyed by cooking.
- Uronic acid, a component of dietary fiber
- Oxalic acid, found in certain fruits and vegetables
- Saturated fats, found in many of our foods
- Alcohol, in any form
- Aluminum, in the form of antacid medication, when taken in excess

It is possible for foods to contain calcium and only be available to the body in limited quantities. The reason is that these foods contain calcium-binding substances called oxalates (found in many green vegetables) or phytates (found in unleavened grain products). Oxalates bind with calcium to produce insoluble salt (calcium oxalate), which *cannot* be absorbed by the body. Spinach, beet greens, chard and rhubarb contain calcium, but they also contain oxalates that bind with calcium and interfere with calcium absorption. The calcium content of these foods should not be counted as part of your daily calcium intake. Cocoa, soybeans, cashews, and kale also contain oxalates.

Many foods that are high in fiber also contain phytate, which inhibits calcium absorption. Wheat bran has been shown to have a significant inhibiting effect.

A secondary contributing factor is stress. Stress removes magnesium from cells and replaces it with calcium from blood and bones. This causes muscles to become tense as our bodies go into their fight-or-flight mode.

Calcium is constantly lost from our bloodstream through urine, sweat, and bowel movements. It is renewed with calcium from the bones. In this process, bones continuously lose calcium. Bone calcium *must* be replaced through dietary intake of calcium and calcium supplements if there is not enough calcium in food.

Our calcium needs change with the aging process. Up until the age of 30 or so, human beings consume more calcium than they lose. Adequate calcium intake during childhood and adolescence is especially important. Later, the body begins to slip into "negative calcium balance," and bones start to lose more calcium than they take up. The loss of too much calcium can lead to decreased bone density and osteoporosis.

Pay attention to foods that cause calcium loss through the urine. You lose calcium daily through the urine. While a certain amount of calcium loss through urine is natural, there is evidence to suggest that this loss is increased by excess consumption of salt and caffeine:

Salt (Sodium) This is the most common cause of calcium loss through the urine. Since over 90% of sodium comes from food rather than table salt, consumption of foods containing salt should be minimized. A common misconception among health practitioners is that excess sodium intake is the cause of high blood pressure. In many cases it is the lack of potassium and not sodium that is the reason. Also, a calcium deficiency is a potential cause for high blood pressure.

Caffeine This is the second most common cause of calcium loss through the urine. Most experts agree that two to three cups of coffee a day are probably not detrimental *provided* that calcium intake (1200 — 1500 mg/day) is adequate. Drink at least one glass of milk for every cup of coffee. However, if more than three cups are consumed in a day drink non-fat milk to avoid consuming increased amounts of saturated fats and cholesterol. Drinking pure water with ionic coral calcium is a much healthier way to offset the negative effects of caffeine. Cancer patients must avoid intake of caffeine and milk!

Flax Oil* Flaxseed contains a phytochemical known as lignan within the cell matrix of its seed. Much of the interest surrounding plant lignans is based on the suspected association between them and the low incidence of breast and colon cancers of those consuming a plant and grain based vegetarian diet. High levels of lignans are present in the blood, urine and feces of these individuals. Flaxseed contains 100-800 times more plant lignans than does its closest competitors, wheat bran, rye, buckwheat, millet, soybeans and oats. Once consumed, lignans found in flaxseed are converted by bacterial action in the colon to mammalian lignans. They are then circulated through the intestinal tract and liver where their action is enhanced. Here mammalian lignans bind with estrogen receptors with results suggesting they may induce the production of a special sex hormone binding compound. This compound known as sex hormone binding globulin (SHBG) regulates estrogen levels by escorting excess estrogen from the body via its eliminative pathways. It should be noted that lignans are thought to be estrogen modulators, balancing estrogen activity with both weak estrogenic and anti-estrogenic abilities. The FDA and the National Cancer Institute as well as several research institutions at the annual convention on Experimental Biology held in New Orleans, LA, presented these and other positive findings.

Dr. Johanna Budwig is Germany's premier biochemist. In addition, Dr. Budwig holds a Ph.D. in Natural Science, has undergone medical training, and was schooled in pharmaceutical science, physics, botany and biology. She is best known for her extensive research on the properties and benefits of flaxseed oil combined with sulphurated proteins in the diet. She has published a number of books on the subject, including *Cancer — A Fat Problem, The Death of the Tumor,* and *True Health Against Arteriosclerosis, Heart Infarction & Cancer.* Dr. Budwig has assisted many seriously ill individuals, even those given up as terminal by orthodox medical practitioners, to regain their health through a simple regimen of nutrition. The basis of Dr. Budwig's program is the use of flaxseed oil blended with low-fat cottage cheese.

In the mid 1950's, Dr. Budwig began her research on the importance of essential fatty acids (linoleic and linolenic) in the diet. Her subsequent discoveries and announcements sparked mixed reactions. While the general public was eager for this vital information, German manufacturers of commercial dietary fats (margarine, hard shortening, vegetable oils) went to extremes to prevent her from publishing her findings. Fortunately, while Dr. Budwig's conclusions were initially met with resistance backed by those with financial stakes in the commercial fats industry, she persisted. Today, Dr. Johanna Budwig is world renowned for her important discoveries on the benefits of flaxseed oil.

The Flaxseed (Linseed) oil diet was originally proposed by Dr. Budwig, in 1951 and recently re-examined by Dr. Dan C. Roehm M.D. FACP (Oncologist and former cardiologist) in 1990. Dr. Roehm claims: "this diet is far and away the most successful anti-cancer diet in the world." Budwig claims that the diet is both a preventative and a curative. She says the *absence of linol-acids* (in the average western diet) *is responsible for the production of oxydase, which induces cancer growth* and is the cause of many other chronic disorders.

The beneficial oxydase ferments are destroyed by heating or boiling oils in foods, and by nitrates used for preserving meat, hot dogs, salami, and sausage. The theory is: the use of oxygen in the organism can be stimulated by protein compounds of sulphuric content, which make oils water-soluble and which is present in cheese, nuts, onion and leek vegetables such as leek, chive, onion and garlic, but especially cottage cheese. Ferments of cell respiration closely connected with the highly unsaturated fatty acids, are also needed for proper oxidation. It is essential to use only unrefined, cold-pressed oils with high linoleic acid content, such as linseed, sunflower, soya, poppy seeds, walnut, and corn oils. Such oil should be consumed together with foods containing the right proteins, otherwise the oils will have the *opposite effect*, causing more harm than good.

Fats-Good and Bad Dr. Budwig is against the use of what she calls "pseudo" fats. In order to extend the shelf life of their products, manufacturers use chemical processes that render their food products harmful to the body. These harmful fats go by a number of names, including "hydrogenated", "partially hydrogenated" and even "polyunsaturated." The chemical processing of fats destroys the vital electron cloud within the fat. Once the electrons have been removed, these fats can no longer bind with oxygen, and they actually become a harmful substance deposited within the body. The heart, for instance, rejects these fats and they end up as inorganic fatty deposits on the heart muscle itself. Chemically processed fats are not water-soluble when bound to protein. They end up blocking circulation, damage heart action, inhibit cell renewal and impede the free flow of blood and lymph fluids. The bioelectrical action in these areas slows down and may become paralyzed. The entire organism shows a measurable loss of electrical energy, which is replenished only by adding active lipids to the diet. These nutritional fats are vital for humans and animals alike.

Science has proven that fats play an important role in the functioning of the entire body. Fats (lipids) are vital for all growth processing, renewal of cells, brain and nerve functions, even for the sensory organs (eyes and ears), and for the body's adjustment to heat, cold and sudden temperature changes. Our energy resources are based on lipid metabolism. To function efficiently, cells require true polyunsaturated, live electron-rich lipids, present in abundance in raw flaxseed oil. True polyunsaturated fats greedily absorb proteins and oxygen and pump them through the system.

Lipids are only water-soluble and free flowing when bound to protein; thus the importance of protein-rich cottage cheese. When high quality, electron-rich fats are combined with proteins, the electrons are protected until the body requires energy. This energy source is then fully and immediately available to the body on demand, as nature intended.

Note: Fat that has not been heated above 96° F. in the form of unsalted raw butter, raw eggs, raw cream, the fat in and on raw meats, no-salt-added raw cheeses, avocados, fresh coconut and stone-pressed olive oil are recommended in Dr. Kelly's Metabolic Medicine's Cancer Cure Diet. These fats are the easiest to digest, assimilate, and utilize and aid the body in binding with toxins and carrying them to the bowels and out of the body.

PROVEN BENEFITS STILL POURING IN

Since Dr. Johanna Budwig's widely publicized findings on the benefits of flaxseed oil have been supported by scientists around the world, numerous studies conducted using flaxseed oil on numerous disorders have shown impressive results, including anti-tumor activity, increased metabolism, greatly boosted immune system, reduced cholesterol levels, normalized blood pressure levels and inhibition of cancer cell growth. Books, research reports, articles and testimonials abound, all touting the healthy benefits achieved by supplementing the diet with organic, raw, cold-pressed flaxseed oil with low-fat cottage cheese. Dr. Budwig's research was based on using the ratio of 2 tablespoons flaxseed oil mixed with one-quarter cup of low fat cottage cheese. This extensive research, leads to the indisputable conclusion: the fact is supplementing a daily diet with flaxseed oil combined with sulphurated proteins could very well be the most important thing a person can do.

Doctor Johanna Budwig's totally natural formula protects against the development of cancer. People all over the world who have been diagnosed with incurable cancer and sent home to die have actually been cured and now lead normal healthy lives. After three decades of research Dr. Budwig, six-time nominee for the Nobel Award, found that the blood of seriously ill cancer patients was, without exception, deficient in certain important essential ingredients, which included substances called phosphatides and lipoproteins. (The blood of a healthy person always contains sufficient quantities of these essential ingredients. However, without these natural ingredients cancer cells grow wild and out of control.)

Blood analysis showed a strange greenish-yellow substance in place of the healthy red oxygen carrying hemoglobin that belongs there. This explained why cancer patients weaken and become anemic. This startling discovery led Dr. Budwig to test her theory. She found that when these missing natural ingredients where replaced over approximately a three month period, tumors gradually receded. The strange greenish elements in the blood were replaced with healthy red blood cells as the phosphatides and lipoproteins almost miraculously reappeared. Weakness and anemia disappeared and life energy was restored. Symptoms of cancer, liver dysfunction and diabetes were completely alleviated. Dr. Budwig then discovered an all-natural way for people to replace those essential ingredients their bodies so desperately needed in their daily diet. By simply eating a combination of just two natural and delicious foods not only can cancer be prevented but in case after case it was actually cured. (These two natural foods, organic flax seed oil & cottage cheese) must be eaten together to be effective since one triggers the properties of the other to be released.)

After more than 10 years of solid clinical application, Dr. Budwig's natural formula has proven successful where many orthodox remedies have failed. Dr. Budwig's formula has been used therapeutically in Europe for prevention of: Cancer, Arteriosclerosis, Strokes, Cardiac Infarction, Heartbeat (irregular), Liver (fatty degeneration), Lungs (reduces bronchial spasms), and Intestines (regulates activity). Stomach Ulcers (normalizes gastric juices), Prostate (hypertrophic), Arthritis (exerts a favorable influence), Eczema (assists all skin diseases), Old age (improves many common afflictions), Brain (strengthens activity), Immune Deficiency Syndromes (multiple sclerosis, autoimmune illnesses)

BUDWIG'S SCIENTIFIC FINDINGS

Her scientific findings have been systematically suppressed by industry, medicine and politics.

All cells need oxygen for living. The oxygen transport agents in the body, Dr. Budwig discovered, are lipoproteins. These are water-soluble compounds produced by the organism, using unsaturated oils and protein. The protein protects the electrons in the unsaturated fat. Venous blood receives these lipoproteins from the lymphatic (drainage) system before it enters the heart, is pumped to the lungs to receive oxygen, then through the arteries to feed the cells. Doctor Budwig also discovered that blood samples from people with cancer, diabetes, and some kinds of liver disease consistently lacked Essential Fatty Acids (EFAs). She noted the following scientific findings:

- Unrefined Flaxseed oil, in practice, inhibits tumor growth and is useful in the natural treatment of cancer
- Essential fatty acids from refined oil help promote tumor growth (due to trans-fats present in *all* American commercial vegetable oil)
- Respiration requires electrons to recover the food energy

- Cell membranes are controlled by surface-active lipoids
- The immune system is governed by bioelectric energies stored in energy reservoirs

The oil/protein ratio in our food is therefore important. Unsaturated oil + protein is an essential food, not a medicine. If cells do not receive enough oxygen and building substances, they start degenerating. "Civilized" food contains many saturated fats with hardening or antioxidant treatments (for longer conservation). They cannot accept oxygen, and are bio-electrically inert, even poisonous. They block the circulation and hinder cell life. In addition we eat too much denatured sugar and proteins (and many other poisons), which prevent normal oxygen circulation. We take too many medications — sleeping pills, narcotics, for example. In reality we are killing ourselves. The consequences are lack of energy, heart insufficiency, infarction, muscle degeneration, diabetes, arteriosclerosis, pneumonia, anemia, dermatosis, and cancer to name some of them. These are *all symptoms* of malnutrition!

About cancer treatment

- Operations increase the frequency of metastases
- Growth-inhibiting irradiations or chemicals do not help, as there is no excessive growth, but degeneration; they only weaken the organism even more
- Statistically there is a clear correlation between the density of doctor population and cancer mortality (Dr. Mittmann)

Dr. Johanna Budwig Mix:
Blender together:

- one (1) cup Organic cottage cheese or yogurt (low fat, not too hard, best make your own)
- two to five (2-5) Tbsp. of flaxseed oil
- one to three (1-3) Tbsp. of freshly ground flaxseed (coffee grinder ($15) works fine)
- enough water to make it soft
- little cayenne

Optional:

- little garlic
- little red pepper
- little champagne

Make it very soft. Eat some of it every day. (Adjust quantities for your taste!) Additional recipes are available at *www.datadepo.com/cancercure/budwig.htm.*

In 1931 Otto Warburg answered one of the questions regarding the primary cause of cancer, that present day research oncologists have been asking. Doctor Warburg discovered the conditions within the cell that were necessary to produce the mutations. The early work of two time Nobel Prize-winner Otto Warburg, some seventy plus years ago, (Cause and prevention of Cancer, Biochem, Zeits, 152: 514-520,1924), showed clearly that cancer was associated with *anaerobic (deficiency of oxygen)* conditions, resulting in *fermentation (production of lactic acid)* and a *marked drop in the pH of the cell* (Low pH Hyperthermia Cancer Therapy; Cancer Chemotherapy Pharmacology 4; 147-145, 1980). Moreover, *the production of mutations cannot occur with the pH of the cell in the healthy calcium buffered 7.4 to 6.6 range,* a range which assures the breakdown of glucose into amino acids that promote healthy DNA synthesis. The DNA (deoxyrbonucleic acid) has the master set of amino acid code, and it uses different kinds of RNA (ribonucleic acid) as messengers to convey its instructions to the protein-making machinery. *M.Von Arenne showed that both high and low pH solutions quickly kill the cell. He was also able to show that when the pH is slightly above the normal pH of 7.4 the toxic enzymes, which characterize the low pH cells are neutralized and the cancer cells will enter a dormant state.* Thus the success of the "caustic solution treatment" (use of an alkaline solution to wash the surgical site where the cancer was removed) of tumors by the turn-of-the-century doctors could now be explained. Also, it should be noted that by definition, alkaline solutions are made up of hydroxyl (oxygen-hydrogen) radicals and, therefore, are oxygen rich. In the absence of oxygen in an acidic intracellular fluid, the glucose undergoes fermentation into lactic acid, causing the pH of the cell to drop even further, thereby inhibiting the production of the four amino acids Adenosine, Cytosine, Guanine and Threonine nucleotides that allow for normal DNA synthesis. This provides the necessary conditions for toxic enzymes to produce radicals that will bond with carcinogens. The complexes they produce will bind with specific sequences of nucleotides in the DNA, causing the template to be altered, thereby setting the scene for the abnormal replication of DNA to trigger cancer.

Thus, in the healthy, calcium buffered, slightly alkaline cell environment, the conditions required for the propagation of cancer do not exist. It remains dormant, or dies. Dr. Reich noted that his cancer patients demonstrated:

- Lifestyle defects responsible for deficiency of calcium and/or vitamin D;
- Symptoms and physical signs of ionic calcium deficiency syndrome; and,
- A greater than normal incidence of these ionic calcium deficiency diseases.

Thus, he concluded cancer is the ultimate adaptation to ionic calcium deficiency, "tailor-made" to survive and to thrive in an ionic calcium deficiency environment. Dr. Reich found that the cancer in many of his patients seemed to go into remission once their calcium deficiency was corrected, by a change of lifestyle including diet and with mineral and vitamin supplements that raised the pH of their cellular fluids. Their associated ionic calcium deficiency diseases were also suppressed.

Doctor Reich's and Warburg's discoveries are crucial to understanding the cause of cancer. However, today we are faced with other overlaying factors, which were not major issues during the period extending from the 1920's to 1960's. These other cancer factors include chemical toxicity of our environment (over 1000 new chemicals are introduced into our environment every year), mercury (72 tons are placed in dental patient's teeth world wide every year) and daily exposure to other heavy metal toxicities (aluminum, cadmium, lead, nickel, etc.), pervasiveness of processed food with all the chemical additives, exposure to geopathic stress (electromagnetic fields that surround our bodies on a daily basis) and psychological distress as witnessed by our fast-paced lives. In addition to the calcium deficiencies and pH (acid) imbalance, these other factors must be evaluated and rectified to resolve the present day cancer scourge.

Another interesting fact is that cancer is virtually unknown to the Hopi Indians of Arizona and the Hunza of northern Pakistan, so long as they stay in the same environment. This strongly suggests that something they are consuming is protecting them from cancer. The only significant difference is their water supply. The Hopi water is rich in rubidium and potassium, and the Hunza water is rich in cesium and potassium, making both of the water supplies rich with very caustically ("capable of destroying or eating away by chemical reaction") active metals. Researchers such as Dr. K. Brewer (The Mechanisms of Carcenogenesis, 1979, Journal of IAPM, Vol., V, No.2) and Dr. H. Sartori found that, by not only addressing the calcium deficiency, but by also using these minerals to raise the pH to above the 7.4 range to a pH of 8.5, the cancer cells would die, while the healthy cells would live, thus once again verifying the observations of both the turn-of-the-century doctors and researchers like Dr. Reich. Both Brewer and Sartori would treat their cancer patients with the salts of both rubidium and cesium. These salts have large and extremely alkaline metal ions that can enter the cells through the large nutrient channels, but like the large potassium ions, they have great difficulty in getting out of the cell due to the small ion cell exit channels. Thus, in this oxygen-rich, alkaline environment, cancer cells die quickly, with no damage to the healthy cells, and therefore no serious side effects. The decomposing cells provide the nutrients for renewed health and normal DNA replication. In his publication, "Cesium Therapy in Cancer Patients," Sartori describes the 2-week treatment of 50 last stage, metastasized, terminal cancer patients (13 comatose), with cesium chloride salts. All were expected to die within weeks, with the survival rate being less than one in ten million. After 2 weeks, 13 died with autopsies showing no presence of cancer. After 12 months, 12 more had died, but 25, or an astounding 50% survived. Unfortunately, cries of quackery and persecution from the medical establishment have driven this caustic cancer therapy research, started by Nobel Prize winner Dr. Otto Warburg, out of mainstream medicine.

Genetic Code The instructions for life are contained in the sequences of bases that make up DNA (deoxyrbonucleic acid) and its sister molecule RNA (ribonucleic acid). The DNA has the master set, and it uses different kinds of RNA as messengers to convey its instructions to the protein-making machinery.

Both DNA and RNA contain combinations of four bases: Adenosine (A), Guanine (G), Threonine (T), and Cytosine (C) in the case of DNA. In RNA the Threonine is replaced by the very similar Uracil (U).

Remembering that there are just 20 amino acids in proteins, the problem biologists faced in the 60's was: how can 4 bases code for 20 proteins: if one base = one amino acid, only four different amino acids could be produced. If the bases were read in twos, there are 16 possible combinations; still not enough. If the bases are read in threes, there are 64 possible combinations. This is too many but it doesn't matter. After much ingenious experimental work it was conclusively proved by the end of the 60's that DNA does code in triplets to make proteins. Some amino acids have no less than 6 different codes that work for them, and three of the codes are not for protein at all: they are stop signals, telling the machinery to end the chain at this point.

The whole apparatus is very similar to a computer software program. The code was established long before the actual mechanism was deduced whereby the amino acids, RNA and the cell machinery are marshaled to carry out the synthesis, and in fact this work is still going on. But the simplicity and elegance of the code means that whenever a protein structure is known the corresponding DNA and RNA structures can be inferred, and vice versa. When the Human Genome Project is completed, the complete DNA sequence for every protein in human beings will be known.

Once the cell environment is severely altered and the DNA mutates and replication goes out of control, heroic measures must swiftly be taken to reverse the process. The following supplements marked with an asterisk were those used as part of the protocol to reverse my wife's stage III ovarian cancer. Those nutrients not marked with an asterisk are presented because they have merit as excellent products for treating cancer. *I cannot emphasize enough the importance of testing each supplement for biocompatibility and dosage with the patient's energy pattern.* There are literally thousands of nutritional products on the market and one can spend a fortune and still not achieve results. Selecting the correct supplements will help restore the quality and quantity of the patient's energy. They also help restore the myriad of functions within the body without damaging the systems of the body and overloading the detoxification mechanism (lymphatics, liver, kidneys, lungs and intestines). This paradigm differs drastically from the allopathic model of strictly trying to "kill" the cancer without body regeneration and regard for the damage inflicted on the host.

Oxygen Elements Plus* Oxygen Elements Plus supplies the body with a steady diet of free oxygen, hydrogen, full spectrum minerals, amino acids, and enzymes — all the while cleansing the body's cells, including the colon.

Oxygen Elements Plus Is:

- a *powerful free radical scavenger.* This is especially noticeable, for example, with patients who use it when they require chemotherapy and/or radiation. These patients report fewer or no side effects, especially nausea, weight loss, and hair loss.

- a *metabolic efficiency catalyst.* This enhances nutrient absorption and increases waste metabolism. Patient's absorb more nutrient value from the foods and supplements they consume, because the trace mineral activated enzymes (both digestive and metabolic enzymes) work more efficiently. The strong catalytic activity of Oxygen Elements Plus allows for dosage reduction with drug therapy and promotes greater nutrient absorption and availability of vitamins, minerals, herbs, and other nutrients.

- an *energy booster.* With the increased energy reserves the Oxygen Elements Plus imparts, there is a gradual but significant detoxification of cellular wastes, allowing the body to function cleanly and efficiently, further increasing energy level over time. The trace element support of the digestive, nervous and endocrine systems' functions may contribute to increased energy, relief from allergies, and decreased sleep requirements.

- a *detoxifier.* Oxygen Elements Plus increases the energy potential in the body. The natural result in most people's bodies is to increase metabolism of waste material out of the body. This can result in detoxification symptoms — headaches, achiness, skin eruptions, recurrence of past symptoms — if it is done too rapidly, and especially if the eliminative channels of the body are congested.

- designed to balance the body's metabolism.

- is *highly charged electrostatically,* and its dibase solution has a bipolar valence, creating a dualistic healing approach to tissue imbalances. This means that whether there is an anabolic or catabolic imbalance, Oxygen Elements Plus creates an appropriate balance and activates the body's rapid healing response.

- a *wound healer.* It acts as a free electron donor, repairing tissue on contact at the cellular level. People using Oxygen Elements Plus topically report very satisfactory results with warts, moles, other skin anomalies, athlete's foot, fingernail and toenail fungus, diabetic ulcers, and skin cancer. It cauterizes and disinfects wounds instantly. Painful paper cuts could heal in hours.

- a *water treatment.* It was first developed in 1956 to make potable water for the military. The powerful bacteriostatic and flocculating effects of Oxygen Elements Plus can be witnessed by adding two drops of Hydroxygen Plus to a gallon of water and setting the mixture aside for four to eight hours. The result is drinkable water.

- *extraordinary.* There is no secret behind the value of trace minerals and micronutrients. The secret of the effectiveness of Oxygen Elements Plus is the physics involved in capturing, combining, and concentrating these elements into one easy-to-take drop in a glass of water. Because the elements in Oxygen Elements Plus are in a special ionic form in colloidal suspension, Oxygen Elements Plus replenishes proper blood levels of these nutrients and enhances the metabolic benefit of other supplements and nutrients, as well as assisting in the elimination of toxins and toxic waste materials from the body.

Disclaimer These statements have not been evaluated by the Food and Drug Administration. These products are not intended to diagnose, treat, cure or prevent any disease. The statements are for informational purposes only and are not meant to replace the services or recommendations of a physician or qualified health care practitioner. Those with health problems or women who are pregnant are advised to consult their physician before taking any nutritional supplement. Available at *www.life-support-nutrition.com.*

Enzymes — OmegaZyme The State of Our Digestion-Understanding the Role of Digestive Enzymes by Jordan Rubin, N.M.D., C.N.C.

According to the Surgeon General's Report on Nutrition and Health, eight out of 10 leading causes of death in the United States are diet related. Digestive problems are the number one health problem in North America. Digestive complaints from hemorrhoids to colon cancer result in more time lost at work, school, and play than any other health-related problem. Many of these digestive problems were rare or non-existent less than a century ago.

Why is this? And how can we return to the health of our ancestors? Consume enzyme-rich foods and "live" enzyme supplements.

A stable supply of all enzymes is essential for the human body, of paramount importance. "Alas, our increasingly toxic eating habits and lifestyle not only deprives us from the enzymes we must import into our body, but also deteriorates the organs in charge of producing the body's own enzymes," notes Dr. Peter R. Rothschild, of the Faculty of Natural Medicine at the Peoples University of the Americas. "The progressive, overall depletion of enzymes leads to a situation in which we can neither digest the food we eat, nor can our body synthesize the materials required for cell repair and maintenance.

Therefore, not only general but also a partial, specific enzyme deficit is unquestionably responsible for many of the diseases that escalate in the wake of our relentlessly deteriorating lifestyle.

"Summing up the situation, the corollary to our increasingly worsening enzyme deficiencies is a progressive failure to digest proteins, fats, sugars, starches and other carbohydrates, which causes a great variety of diseases."

Lymph Gland Blockages It is in the area of lymph gland blockage that the work of Dr. Rothschild truly shines and should grab the attention of both health-conscious consumers and a wide range of health professionals.

"Incompletely digested protein and/or carbohydrate molecules trigger a domino-effect insofar that the fragmentary breakdown compounds produce a secondary carbohydrate-polysaccharides — which condense in the tissue fluids of the body, and combine with excess proteins forming a substance known as mucoproteins", says Dr. Rothschild. "This is an aggregate of undigested proteins, forming long chains of polypeptides that adhere to unassimilated carbohydrates. In a worst-case scenario, mucoproteins can also condense in plasma. *The accretion of mucoprotein is the main cause of lymphatic congestion, which is the foremost trigger factor of a great variety of severe pathologies..."*

The consequences of lymph gland blockages cannot be underestimated. The lymphatic system defends the body from foreign invasion by disease-causing agents such as viruses, bacteria, or fungi. The lymph system contains a network of vessels that assists in circulating body fluids. These vessels transport excess fluids away from interstitial spaces in body tissue and return it to the bloodstream for eventual elimination. Lymphatic vessels prevent the backflow of the lymph fluid. They have specialized bean-shaped organs called lymph nodes that filter out destroyed microorganisms. If the lymph system is malfunctioning, internal toxicity will increase and set the stage for disease.

Why We Need Enzymes Certainly one of the keys to improving health, especially unblocking the lymph system and maintaining healthy immune function in the gut, is to insure an optimal amount of enzyme activity in the body. Enzymes are catalysts in the body, protein-like substances, that help maintain the tissues, orchestrate the many functions of the body, and digest food. Unfortunately food enzymes are destroyed at temperatures above 118° F. Thus, all cooked and processed foods are devoid of food enzymes. Another factor is decreased function of the thyroid gland. The thyroid governs the body's metabolism or burning of food and energy production. A hypo or under function of this gland will cause a lowering of the core temperature of the body and since enzymes are temperature sensitive they will not function properly. In addition fluoride from fluoridated water or toothpastes will suppress thyroid function. To make matters worse, metal fillings in the teeth are comprised of 50 to 60 percent mercury, a poison. It is well documented that mercury fillings leak out 24/7 and are carried from the mouth via the lymphatic system directly to the thyroid. Once in the thyroid, the mercury will bind the iodine, preventing hormone production. These are some of the issues that must be dealt with in order to restore health.

The research of Dr. Edward Howell in the 1930's revealed that people living in "civilized" or industrialized countries had pancreases twice as large as those who consumed primitive diets (raw foods). Consumption of processed foods was responsible for over working the pancreas and decreasing its enzyme production. Doctor Howell was able to resolve many medical problems by supplying his patients with enzymes alone.

Doctor Kelly believes cancer is a disorder of protein metabolism due to inadequate production or utilization of protein-digesting enzymes. He advocates use of pancreatic enzymes between meals to digest the cancer cells. Kelly's approach also involves dietary protocols to support individual metabolic types. Kelly also offers a simple yet profound self-evaluation for determining if the pancreas is functioning properly:

When the pancreas is dysfunctional and fails to produce adequate amounts of amylase (starch digestion), lipase (fat digestion), protease (protein digestion) and other enzymes like trypsin and chymotrypsin, the following symptoms usually occur:

- The first indication of pancreatic failure is indigestion with belching and passing of excessive gas (flatulence). Belching immediately after a meal signifies a gall bladder problem. Flatulence an hour to an hour and a half after meals signifies a lack of pancreatic enzymes.
- The second indication, which occurs over an extended time, is the dental condition called pyorrhea.
- The third indication is focusing problems of the eyes. This occurs because the tiny muscles of the eyes do not take much protein loss to interfere with their function.

Two other factors include halitosis (bad breath) and foul smelling stools. Lack of adequate digestive enzymes allows putrefaction to occur in the stomach and intestines accounting for the odor problems.

If one does not consume proper levels of enzymes from foods or supplements the following symptoms may occur: excessive gas and bloating (particularly after meals), diarrhea and/or constipation, heartburn, low energy, acne, arthritis, allergies, insomnia, high cholesterol and many more.

Once enzymes have completed their appointed task they are destroyed, so there must be a constant replacement of enzymes. The best way to assure the body receives an adequate amount of enzymes every day is to consume a diet high in "live" raw and fermented foods. A high potency, broad-spectrum digestive enzyme supplement such as Omegazyme, DigestEnz or ProactEnz is also essential. Available from: ICNR, Inc. 1-800-272-2323 or order on line at *www.icnr.com.*

Aloe Vera* The Aloe Vera plant produces at least 6 antiseptic agents: Lupeol, salicylic acid, urea nitrogen, cinnamonic acid, phenols, and sulphur. They kill or control mold, bacteria, fungus, and viruses, explaining why the plant has the ability to eliminate many internal and external infections. The Lupeol and salicylic acid in the juice explains why it is a very effective painkiller.

Aloe Vera contains at least three anti-inflammatory fatty acids, cholesterol, campersterol and B-sitosterol (plant sterols) which explains why it is a highly effective treatment for burns, cuts, scrapes, abrasions, allergic reactions, rheumatoid arthritis, rheumatic fever, acid indigestion, ulcers, plus many inflammatory conditions of the digestive system and other internal organs, including the stomach, small intestine, colon, liver, kidney, and pancreas. B-sitosterol is also a powerful anti-cholestromatic, which helps to lower harmful cholesterol levels, helping to explain its many benefits for heart patients.

Since aloe contains at least 23 polypeptides (immune stimulators), we can understand why Aloe juice helps control a broad spectrum of immune system diseases and disorders, including HIV and AIDS. The polypeptides, which are sugars bound to proteins that have a pronounced effect on immune function, plus the anti-tumor agents in Aloe emodin and Aloe lectins, explain its ability to control cancer.

In 1989, Researchers from Okinawa, Japan reported in the Japanese Journal of Cancer Research, that Aloe contained at least three anti-tumor agents, emodin, mannose, and lectin. The researchers concluded that Aloe controls pulmonary carcinogenesis and is effective in the treatment of leukemia and sarcoma and that it would prevent the development of tumors.

In 1994, Dr. Wendell Winters, University of Texas Health Science Center, at San Antonio, reported Aloe contains at least 140 substances including substances, which control cell growth and division, reduce inflammation, stimulate the growth of white cells and other immune-function cells, heal wounds and fight infection. Winters calls Aloe "a pharmacy in a plant."

Aloe Vera from Medi Herb® Aloe Vera Concentrate contains polysaccharides, in particular, acetylated galactomannan (called acemannan). Acemannan has been shown to be a powerful immune stimulant providing anti-cancer and anti-viral effects. This product contains a minimum of 11.25 mg/mL of acemannan to ensure optimal strength and quality. Many other constituents are also present, and together taken internally they:
- support healthy digestive function
- promote a healthy immune response, and
- maintain a healthy blood sugar level when combined with a balanced diet

Although there are more than 300 species of Aloe vera, only four have medicinal value. Aloe contains at least seven superoxide dismutases, compounds with anti-oxidant activity. Animal studies suggest chemopreventive properties for aloe; the juice appears to inhibit cancer-cell division. — Betsy Levy (Hamilton, Rowan. Strengths and Limitations of Aloe Vera. The American Journal of Natural Medicine. December 1998, Vol. 5, No. 10:pp. 30-33.)

Caution: Not to be used during pregnancy and lactation unless otherwise directed by a qualified health care practitioner. Available from: ICNR, Inc. 1-800-272-2323 or order on line at: *www.icnr.com.*

Alpha Lipoic Acid* Several qualities distinguish alpha-lipoic acid from other antioxidants; it has been described at various times as the universal metabolic antioxidant. It neutralizes free radicals in both the fatty and watery regions of cells, in contrast to vitamin C, which is water-soluble and vitamin E, which is fat-soluble.

The body routinely converts some alpha-lipoic acid to dihydrolipoic acid, which appears to be an even more powerful antioxidant. Both forms of lipoic acid quench peroxynitrite radicals, an especially dangerous type consisting of both oxygen and nitrogen, according to a recent paper in FEBS Letters (Whiteman M, et al., FEBS Letters, 1996; 379:74-6). Peroxynitrite radicals play a role in the development of atherosclerosis, lung disease, chronic inflammation, and neurological disorders.

Alpha-lipoic acid also plays an important role in the synergism of antioxidants. It directly recycles and extends the metabolic life spans of vitamin C, glutathione, and coenzyme Q10, and it indirectly renews vitamin E.

An ideal therapeutic antioxidant would fulfill several criteria. These include absorption from the diet, conversion in cells and tissues into a usable form, a variety of antioxidant actions (including interactions with other antioxidants) in both membrane and aqueous phases, and low toxicity." "Alpha-lipoic acid is unique among natural antioxidants in its ability to fulfill all of these requirements making it a potentially highly effective therapeutic agent in a number of conditions in which oxidative damage has been implicated." In regards to cancer, alpha-lipoic acid can inhibit the activation of "nuclear factor kappa-B", a protein complex involved in cancer and the progression of AIDS. (Suzuki YJ, et al., Biochemical & Biophysical Research Communications, 1992;189:1709-15). In addition, recent data shows that alpha-lipoic acid potentiates the cytotoxic effects of Vitamin C toward abnormal cells. Available from: ICNR, Inc. 1-800-272-2323 or order on line at: *www.icnr.com*.

Alterative Compound* This formulae enhances lymphatic, liver and kidney function: Red Clover flower, Burdock Root, Buckthorn bark, Licorice root, Oregon Grape root, Stillingia root, Phytolacca root, Prickly Ash bark, Quassia wood, Potassium iodide.

Suggested dosage This formulation is added to the Herbal C mixture to reduce the number of separate dosages per day. Add entire one fluid ounce bottle to 1.6 quarts (50.7 ounces) of stock Herbal C solution. Warm two ounces of the stock solution mixed with two ounces of spring water. Take three times a day between meals. Martinelli's unfiltered apple juice jars make excellent storage containers for the compound. Available from: ICNR, Inc. 1-800-272-2323 or order on line at: *www.icnr.com*.

Artemisinin* Pure Artemesia annua, an herb from the Far East, has been used for centuries in Chinese medicine for addressing specific intestinal parasites. Pure artemisinin or Qinghaosu, the active constituent of the herb Artemesia annua (sweet wormwood), provides approximately 300 times more of the active constituent artemisinin than the whole herb itself. Research has shown Artemisinin to be particularly beneficial in balancing the microbiology of the GI tract.

Caution: Contraindicated for pregnant or nursing women. Artemisinin produces an oxidizing effect in the stomach and intestines. A healthcare practitioner should monitor long-term administration longer than 2 or 3 months. Combining with antioxidants or iron may decrease effectiveness. Some individuals may experience detoxification reactions. The above statement has not been evaluated by the U.S. Food and Drug Administration. The product is not intended to diagnose, treat, cure, or prevent any disease. Other ingredients: Cellulose, stearic acid. Available from: ICNR, Inc. 1-800-272-2323 or order on line at: *www.icnr.com.*

Black Currant Seed Oil* Black Currant Seed Oil is an excellent source of the omega-6 fatty acids. Gamma-linolenic acid converts to a hormone-like substance called prostaglandin E1 (PGE1). PGE1 helps maintain blood flow, fat metabolism, and fluid balance.

Omega-6 fatty acids are "good fats" and are scientifically proven to promote efficient nutrient utilization needed for cardiovascular growth and development. They also may increase the fluidity or pliability of cell membranes to help keep cells functioning efficiently, which promotes healthy energy and vitality. Omega-6 fatty acids have a number of health benefits including promotion of healthy cholesterol levels, cardiovascular health and cellular health throughout the body. They also provide critical support for the healthy cellular uptake of nutrients and cellular export of waste and metabolites. Available from: ICNR, Inc. 1-800-272-2323 or order on line at: *www.icnr.com.*

Boswellia Complex* Boswellia Complex contains Boswellia resin, Celery Seed, Ginger and Turmeric. These herbs provide many phytochemicals including triterpene acids (especially the boswellic acids), several essential oils (one of which contains terpenes and phthalides), coumarins, flavonoids, pungent principles (including gingerols) and yellow pigments referred to as diarylheptanoids (including curcumin). This tablet contains two herbs with standardized levels of key phytochemicals to ensure optimal strength and quality. The Boswellia component is standardized to contain 180 mg of boswellic acids per tablet, and the Turmeric component contains 70.4 mg/tablet of curcuminoids. These and other unnamed compounds within Boswellia Complex work together to:

- support the normal function of the kidneys to clear acidic waste products effectively
- maintain and support healthy joints
- promote the body's normal resistance function
- support healthy circulation
- support healthy response to environmental stresses, and provide antioxidant protection.

Caution: Not to be used during pregnancy and lactation unless otherwise directed by a qualified health care practitioner. Available from: ICNR, Inc. 1-800-272-2323 or order on line at: *www.icnr.com.*

Carnivora A typical treatment protocol for advanced disease would include daily IV infusions (preferably six days per week) of 12ml diluted in 250ml of .9% NaCl infused over 4 hours. In many *advanced cases, a range of 30ml to 100ml daily* is used for IV infusion. This *escalated dose is diluted in 500ml of .9% NaCl and infused over 4 hours.* For cancer present in the brain, it is essential to use 500ml of 20% Mannitol (for 30ml to 100ml daily administration) as a substitute for Sodium Chloride to allow Carnivora to cross the blood-brain barrier.

The applicable dose will depend on factors such as the condition of the patient, type of disease and the presence and extent of the administration of previous toxic therapies, i.e., chemotherapy, radiation, etc. For advanced disease and to maintain the presence of Carnivora systemically due to it's short lifespan in vivo (approx. 4 hours), the patient must ingest additional Carnivora by either sublingual drops ranging from 120 to 250 drops daily and/or subcutaneous injection of 1ml in the am and 1ml in the pm. Intramuscular injection of 2ml in the am and 2ml in the pm may be a substitute for subcutaneous injection. In most cases, the employment of sublingual drops and/or subcutaneous or i.m. injection is utilized as adjuvant therapy to maintain a particular level of Carnivora in the bloodstream. In earlier stages of disease, both types of injection and sublingual drops may be employed as a primary treatment. It is interesting that former President Ronald Reagan used Carnivora drops to assist in eradicating colon cancer. *It is recommended that the patient take between six and nine 125 mcg. capsules of Carnivora over the course of the day in addition to the ingestion of Carnivora extract.* A variety of supportive nutrients and procedures (enzymes, herbs, glandulars, megavitamins, hormones, herb synergy tea, non-chemotherapeutic pharmaceuticals, hyperthermia, etc.) may be part of the protocol. These nutrients and procedures will be covered in future articles. Finally, Carnivora can be used preventively in oral form. One 125 mcg. capsule taken 3-4 times daily is considered sufficient to boost and enhance immune action assuming dietary and lifestyle factors have been addressed. The sterile product is virtually free of endotoxins and pyrogens (less than 1 nanogram per ml).

Cataplex® B* Standard Process laboratory produces two primary divisions of the B-complex vitamins: Cataplex® B and Cataplex® G; each with complementary actions. Cataplex® B contains different components of the B complex that stimulate the metabolic, cardiovascular, and central and peripheral nervous systems. Cataplex® B is beneficial in several ways. First it assists the liver in detoxifying and neutralizing chemicals. Second, it provides tone to smooth muscles, which is one of the primary causes of constipation. Third, it provides the essential fraction B-4, which supports the electrical conduction for the heart. Fourth, pantothenic acid (B-5) supports normal adrenal function, which is crucial in cancer patients. The adrenal glands are the primary means by which the body deals with emergency issues. This fraction of the B-complex helps metabolize lactic and pyruvic acids, which are two major waste products, which irritate the adrenal glands and prevent sleep. Finally, Cataplex® B assists the pancreas to produce their enzymes, which are crucial to digesting food but more importantly digesting the outer protective covering that cancer cells produce to avoid detection by the body's own immune system.

Other Ingredients: Bovine liver, nutritional yeast, porcine duodenum, beet (root), carrot (root), dried beet (root) juice, choline bitartrate, rice (bran) extract, defatted wheat (germ), bovine adrenal, oat flour, soy bean lecithin, mixed tocopherols, ascorbic acid, manganese lactate, inositol, and riboflavin. Honey, niacinamide, potassium para-aminobenzoate, calcium stearate, arabic gum, cocarboxylase, and pyridoxine hydrochloride. Available from: ICNR, Inc. 1-800-272-2323 or order on line at: *www.icnr.com.*

Cat's Claw Complex* The herbs contained in Cat's Claw Complex are Cat's Claw, Pau d'Arco and Echinacea purpurea root. This combination of herbs contains many compounds including pentacyclic oxindole alkaloids, quinovic acid glycosides, sterols, caffeic acid derivatives (especially cichoric acid), alkylamides and naphthoquinones (especially lapachol).

Other Ingredients: Calcium acid phosphate, cellulose, hypromellose, magnesium stearate, silica, sodium starch glycollate. Together these herbs and the compounds within them help to:

- enhance immune system function
- support respiratory system health
- maintain healthy mucous membranes
- promote healthy response to environmental stresses
- regulate bowel function
- promote healthy bowel flora
- support and maintain healthy blood, and
- provide antioxidant protection.

Caution: Contraindicated in pregnancy and lactation unless otherwise directed by a qualified health care practitioner. Contraindicated in patients taking anticoagulant drugs. Contraindicated in known allergy to plants of the daisy family. These statements have not been evaluated by the Food & Drug Administration. These products are not intended to diagnose, treat, cure or prevent any disease. Available from: ICNR, Inc. 1-800-272-2323 or order on line at: *www.icnr.com.*

Coenzyme Q10 * Dr. Atkins, in his monthly newsletter presented some very valuable information about CoQ10. He states that what is good for the heart may also be good for the breast. New research suggests that Coenzyme Q10, a versatile nutrient known for its ability to protect the cardiovascular system may be able to coax some breast cancers into remission. Thirty-two women with breast cancer took 90 mg of CoQ10 along with high daily doses of antioxidants and essential fatty acids. Statistically, six of the women should have died over the course of the two-year study. Remarkably, though, all lived. Some even got better (Biochemical and Biophysical Research Communications, 1 994; 1 99:1 504-8).

How much better? Six women went into partial remission, and breast tumors disappeared entirely in two women who took 300 mg or more of the enzyme per day. Dr. Knud Lockwood, M.D., of Denmark wrote that until the test of CoQI0, he has "never seen a spontaneous complete regression of a tumor, and has never seen a comparable regression on any conventional anti-tumor therapy." This doctor has treated some 200 cases of breast cancer per year for over 35 years, over 70,000 cases.

Dr. Atkins states that he usually recommends 200 to 400 mg of CoQ10 a day. It's part of his patients' personalized treatment program. Coenzyme Ql0 requires some fat for absorption into the blood stream, so it should be taken with the biggest meal of the day, or as a preparation by Phillips Nutritionals called OptiQ100, in which the CoQ10 is dissolved in soybean oil. (Cancer/woman/ Atkins)[6]

What is CoQ10 ? It is a fat-soluble vitamin-like substance present in every cell of the human body and serves as a coenzyme for several of the key enzymatic steps in the production of energy within the cell. It also functions as an antioxidant. It is present in small amounts in a number of foods and its highest concentration occurs in organ meats like the heart, kidney and liver. It is present also in sardines, mackerel and peanuts. Unfortunately it is difficult to derive an optimum amount of CoQ10 from the foods that we eat. One would have to eat over 7 pounds of peanuts, or 3 pounds of mackerel, or 6 pounds of beef daily to obtain 90 mg of CoQ10, an impossible task[7]. However the body also manufactures CoQ10 but this is a rather complex 17-step process requiring vitamin B2, vitamin B3, vitamin B6, folic acid, vitamin B12, vitamin C, pantothenic acid and several trace minerals. Moreover, as we age, our ability to manufacturer CoQ10 diminishes considerably.

Dr. Folker (the man who identified CoQ10 in 1958) argues that sub optimal nutrient intake is almost universal and as a result there is a secondary impairment in the biosynthesis of this important substance[7]. It would follow then that taking supplemental CoQ10 would be the only way to provide this substance in the quantity that has appeared to be beneficial in reversing disease. Like the vitamins discovered years ago, CoQ10 is an essential element of food that is now used to support sick patients where nutritional depletion and cellular dysfunction are present. Since CoQ10 is essential to optimal function of all cells, it is not surprising to find that a number of diverse disease states respond favorably to CoQ10 supplementation[7].

Dr. Peter Langsjoen, M.D., in his paper on CoQ10, states, "It is reasonable to assume that optimal nutrition (which would include optimal levels of CoQ10) is generally beneficial in any disease state, including cancer."

Extensive research has proven that CoQ10 supplementation has no negative side effects whatsoever. In fact, test subjects reported a higher incidence of side effects with inert placebos than with CoQ10[8]. In addition, CoQ10, which is a prescription drug in Japan, is the most prescribed drug in that country and it is estimated to be taken by over 50 million people daily. Since it did not meet the criteria needed for prescription drug classification in the U.S. it was simply classified as a food substance. Since there is no money to be made from it by the drug companies most doctors were not made aware of it. The beneficial effect of this situation, however, is that it is available in most health food shops at reasonable prices.

CLNZ* It is designed to chelate toxic heavy metals such as mercury, lead, nickel, aluminum and beryllium, as well as some toxic chemicals from the body.

Ingredients: Dandelion Root; Pfaffia; Cinquefoil; Milk Thistle; Mountain Mahogany; Yucca; Vit. E; Wahoo; RNA/DNA Liver Factors; L-Methionine. Available from: ICNR, Inc. 1-800-272-2323 or order on line at: *www.icnr.com.*

Cyruta® Plus* Cyruta® Plus contains several important elements; one of which is the vitamin P complex (bioflavonoids), where rutin and quercetin are members. These factors help to maintain the integrity of the capillary walls. They are vital in their ability to increase the strength of the capillaries and regulate permeability. Dried buckwheat (leaf) juice, buckwheat (seed), bovine adrenal Cytosol™ extract, and oat flour.

Other Ingredients: Honey, ascorbic acid, and calcium stearate. Available from: ICNR, Inc. 1-800-272-2323 or order on line at: *www.icnr.com.*

DMSO* A natural doctor, as a result of one of his recent experiments, stated that DMS0 seems to enhance the power of many therapies, and would be particularly helpful for cancer: It has been shown to enhance the power of chemotherapeutic agents, and when given alone tends to force cancer cells to revert toward normal.

He had a personal experience with DMS0 and cancer having had a basal cell carcinoma on his right ear about the size of a dime. It had been there for six months; surgical removal was standard practice. He mixed some shark cartilage and a little vitamin C with DMS0 into a paste and applied it daily to the lesion on his ear. Within about three and a half weeks it had completely disappeared. As one other doctor commented when he saw the results, "I have never seen a basal cell carcinoma spontaneously disappear."

This form of treatment may be acceptable if the cancer is on or near the surface of the skin, again this is a case study of one, and I can find no other references to this type of treatment. DMSO is difficult to obtain, as it is not available in pharmacies. The only place where I know that it can be obtained is in pet supply houses as it is commonly used for the treatment of sore muscles and arthritis in animals. If you buy it in one of these stores and tell them that it is for use on humans they will probably not sell it to you so you can use your discretion. Ninety-nine percent pure DMSO is also available from a compounding pharmacist. It is mixed with other substances like vitamin C, chemotherapeutic agents and Quinoxide for intravenous infusion. Alternative cancer practitioners use it all the time. DMSO acts as a carrier taking substances through cell walls into the interior where their action is critical.

Garlic* Twenty-two studies referenced in the article, Nagourney, RA. Garlic: Medicinal Food or Nutritious Medicine?. Journal of Medicinal Food. February 8, 1999, demonstrate garlic's antibacterial, antifungal, and antiviral properties. Some of these studies indicate garlic's activity against Mycobacterium avium, Pneumocystis carinii, cytomegalovirus, and herpes simplex types I and II, common opportunistic infections in patients with HIV.

Garlic's effect on atherosclerosis is attributed to its ability to dissolve fibrin (a component of blood clots), inhibit platelet aggregation (also responsible for blood clot formation), and lower serum lipids like cholesterol. Garlic increases HDL (high density or "good cholesterol") and lowers LDL (low density or "bad cholesterol") and triglycerides (fats found in serum). One meta-analysis of 28 clinical trials concluded that consumption of one garlic clove a day could reduce serum lipids by nine percent.

Epidemiological studies have found significantly fewer cases of gastric and colon cancers in populations that regularly consume garlic when compared with populations that do not. Over 29 studies demonstrate the ability of different chemical constituents of garlic to inhibit tumor initiation and promotion, induce enzymes that alter carcinogens in food or toxic substances, as well as alter mutagenic agents directly (mutagens alter cellular DNA which can lead to cancer). One animal study found that garlic increased the life span of mice given a lethal dose of cyclophosphamide (a chemotherapeutic agent used in the treatment of cancer) by 70 percent, without disturbing the medication's antitumor effect. Another animal study found a reduction in hair loss and toxicity to cells of the urinary tract in animals first treated with a component of garlic and then treated with cyclophosphamide. These studies indicate that garlic may play a significant role in the treatment as well as the prevention of cancer. Garlic also exhibits free radical scavenging activity, which may help prevent cellular degeneration in the aging process.

The author concludes that all of the benefits of garlic are found in its fresh, natural state. According to this author, highly processed garlic products may not yield allicin and its byproducts. — Leela Devi, MSN, RN. Available from: ICNR, Inc. 1-800-272-2323 or order on line at: *www.icnr.com.*

Grape Seed Extract* This product provides a special fraction of the bioflavonoid group, which has been shown to be a potent antioxidant and may also display metal-binding activity, a property, which may contribute to their antioxidant effects. They also function as an effective anti-inflammatory agent and help potentiate vitamin C and E.

A patented extract of the flavanol proanthocyanidins (PAC) is prepared from grape seeds. These are the most potent of the available proanthocyanidin extracts, having a higher total content of PAC (92%). The proanthocyanidins from grape seeds were discovered and patented by the same researcher who discovered the pine bark extract, and have been well studied analytically, biochemically, toxicologically, and clinically. PAC is a powerful antioxidant due to the component diphenols and related structures. The proanthocyanidin flavonoids offer an excellent option for adjunct nutritional support of small vessel circulation. Due to their superior water solubility, they are absorbed well and are generally well tolerated. Available from: ICNR, Inc. 1-800-272-2323 or order on line at: *www.icnr.com.*

Glutathione* This tripeptide sulfur bearing amino acid is a crucial nutrient for detoxifying the liver. Since the liver is the main organ that filters the blood from the intestine, many potentially dangerous chemicals, heavy metals, molds and other pathogens pass through and must be processed. Some substances become carcinogenic, that is cancer producing, as a result of biotransformation. The process of biotransformation breaks down compounds for phase II detoxification and removal. Some of the breakdown products are carcinogenic and can initiate or increase the toxicity of existing tissues to enhance the growth of cancer. Glutathione is a chelater or grabs on to heavy metals and carries them out of the body via the bile and feces. It is also beneficial in scavenging free radicals, chemical and toxic wastes.

The glutathione levels in our cells are predictive of how long we will live. There are very few other factors, which are as predictive of our life expectancy as our level of cellular glutathione. Glutathione has been called the "master antioxidant", and regulates the actions of lesser antioxidants such as vitamin C, and vitamin E within the body. "We literally cannot survive without this antioxidant," Earl Mindell, R.Ph., Ph.D. *"What You Should Know about the Super Antioxidant Miracle"*

- "Without glutathione, other important antioxidants such as vitamins C and E cannot do their job adequately to protect your body against disease." *Breakthrough in Cell Defense*, Allan Somersall, Ph.D., M.D., and Gustavo Bounous, M.D. FRCS©

- "No other antioxidant is as important to overall health as glutathione. It is the regulator and regenerator of immune cells and the most valuable detoxifying agent in the human body. Low levels are associated with hepatic dysfunction, immune dysfunction, cardiac disease, premature aging, and death." *The Immune System Cure*, Lorna R. Vanderhaeghe & Patrick J.D. Bouic, Ph.D.

- *Glutathione* (L-gammaglutamyl-L-cysteinylglycine) is a tri-peptide of the amino acids cysteine, glycine, and glutamic acid. Glutathione is an antioxidant compound found in living animal and plant tissue. It takes up and gives off hydrogen and is important in cellular respiration. A deficiency of glutathione can cause hemolysis (destruction of red blood cells, leading to anemia) and oxidative stress. Glutathione is essential in intermediary metabolism as a donor of sulfhydryl groups, which are essential for the *detoxification* of acetaminophen. (PDR Medical Dictionary. Spraycar. 1999) Selenium is a structural component of, and a co-factor for, the antioxidant enzyme glutathione peroxidase.

Glutathione is the major internal antioxidant produced by the cell. Glutathione participates directly in the neutralization of free radicals, reactive oxygen compounds, and maintains exogenous antioxidants such as vitamins C and E in their reduced (active) forms. In addition, through direct conjugation, glutathione plays a role in the *detoxification* of many xenobiotics (foreign compounds) both organic and inorganic. Glutathione is an essential component of the human immune response. Proposed mechanisms of immune enhancement include:

- Optimizing macrophage functions
- Offsetting oxidative damage associated with lymphocyte monoclonal expansion
- Stabilizing the mitochondrial membrane thereby, reducing apoptosis (cell death) of lymphocytes

In addition to taking glutathione orally, it can be administered by intravenous push. A trained physician or nurse injects 400mg to 1000mg of glutathione solution rapidly into a vein. This approach enhances chelation or binding of heavy metals and toxins for rapid removal.

Cysteine is a sulfur-containing (sulfhydryl) amino acid, which is present in many proteins, and is in the same class as methionine. Because it is a sulfur-based amino acid, cysteine acts as an antioxidant in the body. Cysteine is an important source of sulfur in human metabolism, and although it is classified as a non-essential amino acid, cysteine may be essential for infants, and may at some point be recognized as an essential or conditionally essential amino acid. The systemic availability of oral glutathione is negligible; the vast majority of it must be manufactured intracellularly. Glutathione (GSH) is a tripeptide made up of the three amino acids cysteine, glycine and glutamate. Glutamate and glycine are readily available in most North American diets, but the amount of cysteine available limit the synthesis of glutathione within the cell. It is the sulfhydryl (thiol) group (SH) of cysteine that serves as proton-donor and is responsible for the biological activity of glutathione.

Some nutritionists advocate the use of *N-acetyl-L-cysteine (NAC)* to provide the precursor for the production of glutathione. NAC is an amine protected version of cysteine that is rapidly hydrolyzed in the body to the amino acid cysteine. (Cysteine is the monomer amino acid). The down side is that NAC supplements are moderately effective, but dosing is limited due to toxic side effects (headache, dizziness, blurred vision) associated with cysteine supplementation.

The free amino acid cysteine is not an ideal delivery system to the cell. It is potentially toxic and is spontaneously catabolized in the gastrointestinal tract and blood plasma. Conversely, cysteine absorbed during digestion as *cystine* (two cysteine molecules linked by a disulfide bond) in the gastrointestinal tract is more stable than the free amino acid cysteine. The disulfide bond is pepsin and trypsin-resistant, but may be split by heat, low pH, and mechanical stress. Cystine travels safely through the GI tract and blood plasma and is promptly reduced to two cysteine molecules upon cell entry.

Cystine is the preferred form of cysteine for the synthesis of glutathione in macrophages and astrocytes. Lymphocytes and neurons prefer cysteine for glutathione production. Optimizing glutathione levels in macrophages and astrocytes with cystine allows these cells to provide cysteine to lymphocytes and neurons directly upon demand.

As an antioxidant, glutathione is essential for allowing lymphocytes to express their full potential, without being hampered by oxyradical accumulation during the oxygen requiring development of the immune response. In a similar fashion, GSH delays the muscular fatigue induced by oxyradicals during the aerobic phase of strenuous muscular contraction. As a detoxification agent, glutathione has been demonstrated to be effective against a number of xenobiotics, including chemical pollutants, various carcinogens and ultraviolet radiation.

Glutathione is a tightly regulated intracellular constituent and is limited in its production by negative feedback inhibition of its own synthesis through the enzyme gamma-glutamylcysteine synthetase, thus greatly minimizing any possibility of over dosage. (source: Physician's Desk Reference for Prescription Drugs (PDR) 2001, p. 1563). Available from: ICNR, Inc. 1-800-272-2323 or order on line at: *www.icnr.com*.

Mistletoe extracts are prepared as aqueous solutions or solutions of water and alcohol, fermented or unfermented. (6,28,34,67,68, reviewed in 52,53) For example, Iscador is an aqueous extract of Viscum album L. that is available in both fermented and unfermented forms. In addition, Iscador products can be subdivided according to the species of host tree. Iscador-M is obtained from apple trees, Iscador-P comes from pine trees, Iscador-Q comes from oak trees, and Iscador-U comes from elm trees. Helixor is an unfermented aqueous extract of Viscum album L., with Helixor-A from spruce trees; Helixor-M comes from apple trees, and Helixor-P from pine trees. Helixor is reported to be standardized by its biologic effect on human leukemia cells grown in the laboratory.(69) Eurixor is an unfermented aqueous extract of Viscum album L. obtained from poplar trees. As indicated previously, there are several potentially active components in mistletoe, and some researchers contend the formulation of mistletoe extracts should vary according to the type of tumor, patient gender and the method of administration. (69,70, reviewed in 53). In modern studies, mistletoe extracts have been administered by intramuscular injection, subcutaneous injection (sometimes in the vicinity of a tumor), or intravenous infusion.

Adverse Effects Although numerous formulations of mistletoe have been used in human studies, the associated side effects have been minimal and non-life threatening. Common side effects found with mistletoe-product injection include soreness and inflammation at the injection site, headache, fever, and chills. (reviewed in 53). Seizures, slowing of the heart rate, abnormally high blood pressure, abnormally low blood pressure, vomiting, and death have been reported after ingestion of mistletoe plants and berries. (reviewed in 53,101) The severity of the toxic effects associated with mistletoe ingestion may depend on the amount consumed and the type of mistletoe plant. (reviewed in 101)

MSM (Methyl Sulfonyl Methane)* Methyl Sulfonyl Methane is a nutrient. Sulfonyl sulfur is found in plants, meats, dairy products and vegetation. MSM is the third largest ingredient in the body. Sulfonyl is a natural sulfa form and part of the sulfur family; it is nutritional, and can't be allergic. It is a normal metabolite of dimethylsulfoxide, better known as DMSO. When taken in its purest form (100% pure), MSM supplements are no more toxic than water. Any excess Methyl Sulfonyl Methane in the system will stay in the blood stream for 12 hours removing toxins and cleaning the interior walls of arteries. It is suggested that vitamin C be taken along with Methyl Sulfonyl Methane. The two work synergistically to help build healthy cells. MSM is a great antioxidant, and it helps to eliminate many unwanted substances from the body by enhancing cellular permeability.

MSM scavenges free radicals, relieves allergies to foods and pollens, and helps the liver produce choline, controls acidity in stomach and ulcers, coats the intestinal tract so parasites lose the ability to hang on, helps with hypersensitivity to drugs, increases the body's ability to produce insulin, is important for carbohydrate metabolism, and speeds wound healing. It is estimated that the human body uses up to about 1/8 tsp. of MSM each day. It needs to be replaced on a regular basis. Good health practices involve replacing essential substances that we naturally use up or lose through illness or abuse. For general use, MSM should be taken internally as a food supplement.

Sulfur is necessary for collagen synthesis. Collagen is an insoluble fibrous protein found in vertebrates (having a backbone or spinal column) as the dominant component of connective tissue fibrils and bones. Sulfur operates as synthesizer and activator with the B vitamins, thiamin, vitamin C, biotin and pantothenic acid, which are needed for metabolism and healthy nerves.

Detoxification One in five may experience negative detoxification symptoms in the first 10 days during which toxins are flushed from the system. Symptoms may include diarrhea, skin rash and/or possible headache along with several days of fatigue. In general the more intense the symptoms, the more toxins there are in the body, and the more MSM is needed for detoxification. To reduce toxic symptoms (if you suspect Candida, chemicals or metals) start with a lower amount of 750 mg, two times a day and build up to 2,000 mg. (four (4) capsules) twice a day. After initial use, energy levels should increase. Available from: ICNR, Inc. 1-800-272-2323 or order on line at: *www.icnr.com.*

Quercetin (Pain Guard Forte™)* PERQUE Pain Guard Forte contains non-citrus bioflavonoid and flavanol mix. Bioflavonoids have long been associated with the synergy they bring to vitamin

C absorption and retention. It has been demonstrated that the flavonoid quercetin (3,3',4',5-7-pentahydroxyflavone) (Q) inhibits the growth of several cancer cell lines and that the antiproliferative activity of this substance is mediated by a so-called type II estrogen binding site (type II EBS). *Scambia G, Ranelletti FO, Benedetti Panici P, et al. Synergistic antiproliferative activity of quercetin and cisplatin on ovarian cancer cell growth. Anticancer Drugs (ENGLAND) , 1:45-48; 1990.*

Quercetin, a phytochemical found in apples, has an even stronger anticancer activity than vitamin C. Phytochemicals, such as flavonoids and polyphenols, are plant chemicals that contain protective, disease-preventing compounds. The flavonoid of Quercetin dihydrate is mixed with OPC 85+, (grape seed derived proanthocyanidins) a flavanol to create a powerful tool that is anti-inflammatory, anti-oxidant, and anti-histamine. Quercetin is useful for those suffering from allergies and swelling due to injury. It may replace conventional allergy pills and anti-histamines and rebuilds intestinal tissue.

This bioflavonoid has been shown to alter gene expression (inducing apoptosis-cell death), and reduce free radical damage and inflammation. Further studies indicate that Vitamin C enhances the cytotoxic effects of Quercetin. Available from: ICNR, Inc. 1-800-272-2323 or order on line at: *www.icnr.com.*

Vitamin C* is a dietary supplement with many health related effects. In some cases, the benefits of Vitamin C without preservatives are best achieved with large concentrations administered intravenously. Vitamin C has several important functions including the synthesis of amino acids and collagen, wound healing, metabolism of iron, lipids and cholesterol. "In particular, vitamin C is a well known anti-oxidant that scavenges free radicals and protects against oxidative DNA damage." An anti-oxidant is one of many chemicals that reduce or prevent oxidation, thus preventing cell and tissue damage from free radicals in the body. Since vitamin C is a six-carbon sugar, it is readily absorbed into cancer cells where it inhibits the carcinogenic effects of hydrogen peroxide on intercellular communication. Until this finding, the mechanism for vitamin C's inhibitory effects on carcinogenic tumor formation was not understood. (C.Y. Lee, Cornell professor of food science and technology, and his South Korean colleagues, Ki Won Lee, Hyong Joo Lee and Kyung-Sun Kang, found the connection.)

Vitamin K is essential for clot formation and liver function. A synthetic form of vitamin K, vitamin K3, has been found to induce cytotoxicity of abnormal cells *in vitro* and *in vivo* and increase the effectiveness and reduce the toxicity of some drugs. Both vitamin C and vitamin K3 exhibit health related effects. Together, vitamin K3 and vitamin C act synergistically.

ProactEnz™* This proprietary blend of protease, substance, which digests protein, has been documented to bind to a macroglobulin that circulates in the blood. Once bound it transforms into a more active form ("fast" alpha 2-macroglobulin) and modulates the action of cytokines (proteins that cause inflammation) and breaks down fibrin. Both actions are critical in resolving inflammation, thrombosis (clots) and wound healing. From a cancer perspective, ProactEnz™, when taken on an empty stomach (two capsules upon arising and two before bedtime), gets into the tissues and helps break down the outer protective protein covering produced by cancer cells to avoid detection by the body's immune system. This process is key to all cancer therapy! This product is only available through health care practitioners. Available from: ICNR, Inc. 1-800-272-2323 or order on line at: *www.icnr.com*.

Wobenzym® N* This systemic enzyme formula has a unique characteristic. Its German manufacturer, Mucos Pharma GmbH, developed a special coating that enables the digestive enzymes to pass through the stomach acids without being dissolved. Only when the product enters an alkaline environment such as the small intestine will it start to breakdown. This feature allows the proteolytic enzymes and especially the Chymotrypsin (a key enzyme in the formula) to remain intact for absorption into the bloodstream where it is carried to the sites of the cancer. Its prime objective is to dissolve the outer protective protein covering of the cancer cells exposing them to the body's immune system for destruction. To be maximally effective, Wobenzym® N must be taken every four hours without food until the cancer is resolved. No matter what cancer protocol one is on this product must be included! Available from: ICNR, Inc. 1-800-272-2323 or order on line at: *www.icnr.com*.

DigestEnz™* This general enzyme formula provides 652mg of a combination of protease, amylase, lipase, CereCalase Plus, Glucoamylase, Malt Diastase, alpha-Galactosidase, Invertase, Lactase, Pectinase and Cellulase. This special blend makes it an effective digestive enzyme product that must be taken with each meal (two capsules). The above three enzyme products are a must for successful cancer treatment. Available from: ICNR, Inc. 1-800-272-2323 or order on line at: *www.icnr.com*.

Rhodiola rosea In a study by O.M. Duhan and colleagues[4], the anti-mutagenic activities of Panax Ginseng and of Rhodiola rosea were compared. It became clear that the extracts of Rhodiola rosea had a higher capacity to counteract gene mutations induced by various mutagens (up to about 90% inhibition in some cases). In addition, Rhodiola rosea is five times less toxic than Panax ginseng. In an experiment on rats with Pliss lymphosarcoma (PLS) it was shown[5] that partial hepatectomy, a course of Rhodiola rosea extract or combined effects inhibit the growth of tumors by 37%, 39% and 59%, respectively, and that of metastases by 42%, 50% and 75%. In one human study[6] oral administration of Rhodiola rosea extract to 12 patients with superficial bladder carcinoma improved the characteristics of the urothelial tissue integration and T-cell immunity. The average frequency of relapses for these patients was found to fall twice.

Rhodiola rosea extracts significantly reduce the yield of cells with the chromosome aberrations in vivo and inhibit unscheduled DNA synthesis induced by N-nitroso-N-methylurea in vitro[7]. It is emphasized that Rhodiola rosea extracts have rejuvenative properties due to their ability to raise the efficiency of the intracellular DNA repair mechanism.

Rhodiola rosea and immunity Rhodiola rosea stimulates the immune system in two ways:
- by specific direct stimulation of immune defense (stimulates one of the most important type of immune cells — Natural Killer Cells, NK-Cells seek and destroy infected cells in our body). Rhodiola rosea normalizes the immune system by improving T-cell immunity.[6] Rhodiola has been shown to increase the body's resistance to toxins that may accumulate during the development of infection.
- by making a person less susceptible to stress. Scientists found out that stress suppresses immunity and destroys our resistance to various forms of bacterial or virus attack. Due to the natural killer cell's effect on tumors Rhodiola rosea may enhance B cell immunity by preventing the suppression of B cell immunity, when taken during periods of stress. Under stress, a great portion of the body's energy is wasted. Chronic exposure to stress continually robs energy from other systems; the general effect is a lowered immune response and decreased health.

My clinical experience, using Optygen™, a Rhodiola rosea based product (which also includes chromium, cordyceps, potassium, sodium, calcium pyruvate and adenosine in its formula), with patients with weak adrenal glands has achieved remarkable results in helping restore lost energy. In my opinion, Optygen™ is the optimum formula available. Recommended dosage for cancer patients is one capsule three times a day. Available from: ICNR, Inc. 1-800-272-2323 or order on line at: *www.icnr.com*.

Selenium is a potent antioxidant that makes vitamin C more effective. Selenium is also required for optimal functioning of the immune system. Selenium is a natural component of wheat germ oil, which also supplies vitamin E, seven tocopherols and essential fatty acids. When ever possible, take vitamins in their natural form, because, they provide synergistic factors that make them work more efficiently. Available from: ICNR, Inc. 1-800-272-2323 or order on line at: *www.icnr.com*.

Transfer Factor Plus™* An independent study using 4Life Transfer Factor™ and Transfer Factor Plus™ yielded unprecedented results in a study done by the Institute of Longevity Medicine in California, a laboratory recognized for its research and expertise in measuring the ability of ingredients to significantly boost the immune system.

4Life Transfer Factor™ and Transfer Factor Plus™ were tested for their ability to increase Natural Killer Cell (NK) activity. The researchers used peripheral blood mononuclear cells (PBMC) isolated from human volunteers. Test results showed that 4Life Transfer Factor™ boosted NK cell activity 103% above normal immune response without supplementation, more than two times higher than the next highest product. The study also showed that Transfer Factor Plus™ increased the NK cell activity 248% above normal immune response without supplementation, or about five times higher than any of the other previously tested products.

Synergistic components of Transfer Factor Plus™ include: IP6®, Cordyceps, Maitake and Shiitake mushrooms, 1,3 Beta Glucans, Aloe, Thymus factor, colostrums. Available from: ICNR, Inc. 1-800-272-2323 or order on line at: *www.icnr.com.*

Ukrain Combining chemotherapy with Ukrain in the advanced stage of ovarian cancer has shown that Ukrain carried on to complete remission, greatly reduced adverse reactions of two cytostatic agents and protected against the spread of metastases.

The first course of Ukrain was started postoperatively: two ampoules i.v. every second day (total 10 injections). Then chemotherapy was performed with Endoxan and Cisplatin with the following schema: the first day 1h Endoxan i.v.; the second day after one-liter kidney protection infusion 12 h Cisplatin i.v. and then one-liter kidney protection infusion. After 10 days rest the next Ukrain course was performed, with chemotherapy with Endean and Cisplatin (as described). Six courses of chemotherapy with Ukrain therapy were performed. After chemotherapy, two courses of Ukrain were performed. Conservative therapy with Ukrain will be given for the next two years without chemotherapy.

Wheat grass juice* Wheat grass juice is extracted from red wheatberry seed sprouts. This strain of wheat has been used worldwide for thousands of years for its healing properties. The juice from wheat grass is high in chlorophyll, active enzymes, vitamins and other important nutrients. Wheat grass is quite possibly the closest thing to the fountain of youth. When consumed, wheat grass juice has been documented to have the following health benefits.

Enzymes Aid In Prevention and Cure of Cancer. Wheat grass has a high concentration of active enzymes. According to an article in the Journal of Longevity Research Vol.2/No.4 1996 by Carol Uebelacker, M.D. enzymes have the ability to combat cancer. In short enzymes dissolve the outer protective covering secreted by the cancer cells and expose them to the immune system for destruction.

Wheat grass Juice Medical Benefits
- Increases hemoglobin production
- Rebuilds and purifies the blood stream
- Improves the body's ability to heal wounds
- Creates an unfavorable environment for unfriendly bacterial growth
- Removes drug deposits from the body

- Neutralizes toxins and carcinogens in the body
- Helps purify the liver
- Improves blood sugar disorders
- Improves digestion
- Removes heavy metals from the body
- Aids in the prevention and curing of cancer

Suggested dosage: one ounce of fresh juice upon arising or seven (7) tablets of Pines wheat grass tablets with water.

Brands:

- Pines International, Inc. 1-800-697-4637 or *www.wheatgrass.com*
- Wild Oats (health food market): purchase flats of fresh living wheat grass.
- Grow your own wheat grass from red wheat berries.

TUMOR MARKERS

Tumor markers are substances that can often be detected in higher-than-normal amounts in the blood, urine, or body tissues of some patients with certain types of cancer. Tumor markers are produced either by the tumor itself or by the body in response to the presence of cancer or certain benign (non-cancerous) conditions.

Measurements of tumor marker levels can be useful — when used along with CAT scans or other tests — in the detection and diagnosis of some types of cancer. However, measurements of tumor marker levels alone are *not* sufficient to diagnose cancer for the following reasons:

- Tumor marker levels can be elevated in people with benign conditions.
- Tumor marker levels are not elevated in every person with cancer — especially in the early stages of the disease.
- Many tumor markers are not specific to a particular type of cancer; the level of a tumor marker can be raised by more than one type of cancer.

In addition to their role in cancer diagnosis, some tumor marker levels are measured before treatment to help doctors plan appropriate therapy. In some types of cancer, tumor marker levels reflect the extent (stage) of the disease and can be useful in predicting how well the disease will respond to treatment. Tumor marker levels may also be measured during treatment to monitor a patient's response to therapy. A decrease or return to normal in the level of a tumor marker may indicate that the cancer has responded favorably to therapy. If the tumor marker level rises, it may indicate that the cancer is growing. Finally, measurements of tumor marker levels may be used after treatment has ended as a part of follow-up care to check for recurrence.

The primary use of tumor markers is to monitor the course of the cancer, patient response to treatment, and disease recurrence. These markers provide a base line for patient and physician to assess the efficacy of treatment. The intent of this information is to provide some of the more frequently used tests for monitoring cancer. This is only a partial list of tumor markers, with enough information to intelligently discuss with a physician a patient's progress during cancer treatment and follow-up status.

Cancer Antigen 125 or CA — 125* *Clinical Significance:* CA 125 is produced by a variety of cells, but particularly by ovarian cancer cells. Studies have shown that many women with ovarian cancer have elevated CA 125 levels. CA 125 is used primarily in the management of treatment for ovarian cancer. In women with ovarian cancer being treated with chemotherapy, a falling CA 125 level generally indicates that the cancer is responding to treatment. Increasing CA 125 levels during or after treatment, on the other hand, may suggest that the cancer is not responding to therapy or that some cancer cells remain in the body. Doctors may also use CA 125 levels to monitor patients for recurrence of ovarian cancer.

Not all women with elevated CA 125 levels have ovarian cancer. Cancers of the uterus, cervix, pancreas, liver, colon, breast, lung, and digestive tract may also elevate CA 125 levels. Non-cancerous conditions that can cause elevated CA 125 levels include endometriosis, pelvic inflammatory disease, peritonitis, pancreatitis, liver disease, and any condition that inflames the pleura (the tissue that surrounds the lungs and lines the chest cavity). Menstruation and pregnancy can also cause an increase in CA 125.

The CA 125 assay is to be used as an aid in monitoring response to therapy for patients with epithelial ovarian cancer. Serial testing for patient CA 125 values should be used in conjunction with other clinical methods for monitoring ovarian cancer. The presence of significant levels of CA 125 has been reported to correlate with disease progression or regression in 80-90% of cases. Persistent elevation in the face of chemotherapy is a poor prognostic sign.

CA 125 is not a good screening tool for ovarian cancer, because it is quite nonspecific. Conditions such as endometriosis, normal pregnancy, pelvic inflammatory disease, uterine fibroids, hepatitis, pancreatitis and cirrhosis may contribute to elevated levels of serum CA 125. Malignancies of breast, lung, and gastrointestinal tract may also be associated with an elevation of this tumor marker.

Reference Range: 0-35 or 0-20 U/mL — depending which lab does the analysis

CA 15-3 Cancers of the ovary, lung, and prostate may also raise CA 15-3 levels. Elevated levels of CA 15-3 may be associated with non-cancerous conditions, such as benign breast or ovarian disease, endometriosis, pelvic inflammatory disease, and hepatitis. Pregnancy and lactation can also cause CA 15-3 levels to rise.

CA 27-29 levels can also be elevated by cancers of the colon, stomach, kidney, lung, ovary, pancreas, uterus, and liver. First trimester pregnancy, endometriosis, ovarian cysts, benign breast disease, kidney disease, and liver disease are non-cancerous conditions that can also elevate CA 27-29 levels.

LASA-P: Lipid Associated Sialic Acid in Plasma (LASA-P)* *Clinical Significance:* Lipid-bound sialic acid (LASA) is considered a tumor marker that lacks the specificity and sensitivity needed for routine tumor detection and diagnosis. But when utilized in conjunction with other tumor markers, it may be useful in identifying selected cancer patients. Elevated concentrations of sialic acid often reflect the release and accumulation of sialyl compounds from malignant cells. Elevations are also noted in inflammatory disorders and in any circumstance associated with significant tissue necrosis. In cancer patients, elevated results can be from the tumor cell surfaces as well as the non-specific inflammatory responses associated with the malignancy.

 Reference Interval: 0-20 mg/dL Some laboratories use a broader range 10-24mg/dL while others use a narrower one 15-20 mg/dL (Dianon)

Cancer Antigen-Breast (CA 15-3)

Clinical Significance: CA-BR is a sensitive marker useful in monitoring the clinical course of breast cancer patients. Whereas elevated levels are only present in a small percentage of patients with localized disease, two-thirds of cases with metastatic disease will have significantly elevated levels. It may also be elevated in patients with hepatitis, cirrhosis, sarcoidosis, tuberculosis, and systemic lupus erythematosus (SLE), as well as in other malignancies (e.g., pancreas, lung, ovary, colon, and liver). Assessments following therapy correlate well with disease progression. Because of relatively low sensitivity and a lack of specificity, CA-BR should not be used as a screening test.

 Reference Range: 0-31 U/mL

Cancer Antigen-GI (CA 19-9) *Clinical Significance:* Cancer antigen-GI (CA-GI) is of clinical use because it is expressed, at high levels, in most patients with carcinomas of the pancreas, liver, biliary tract, stomach, colon, and breast. As with other tumor markers, it is of little use in screening, but valuable in monitoring for disease progression in established cases. The specificity of CA-GI is limited by its expression in patients with pancreatitis and inflammatory gastrointestinal diseases. CA-GI and carcinoembryonic antigen (CEA) may be used together to help differentiate benign disease from pancreatic carcinoma.

 Reference Range: 0-37 U/mL

 Note: This test uses a kit designated by the manufacturer as "for research use, not for clinical use." The performance characteristics of this test were validated by ARUP Laboratories,

Inc. The U.S. Food and Drug Administration (FDA) has not approved this test. The results are not intended to be used as the sole means for clinical diagnosis or patient management decisions. ARUP is authorized under Clinical Laboratory Improvement Amendments (CLIA) and by all states to perform high-complexity testing.

Cytomegalovirus (CMV) *Clinical Significance:* CMV infections in humans are widespread. Infection of normal children and adults usually results in asymptomatic disease, but the infection can cause hepatitis, pneumonia, or a mononucleosis-like illness. CMV infection is frequent and severe in patients with defects in cellular immunity, such as those with acquired immunodeficiency syndrome (AIDS), recipients of organ transplants, or *cancer patients*. An important primary source of virus is blood transfusions. Seronegative individuals transfused with blood from seropositive donors have a high risk of developing CMV infection. Thus, serologic testing for CMV is important in screening blood for transfusion to neonates or to immunocompromised patients. Serologic testing for CMV is also included in pregnancy screening tests and as an aid in diagnosing active or recently acquired CMV infections likely to be acquired by the fetus.

A significant increase in IgG antibody suggests, but does not confirm, recent infection. In immunocompromised patients, IgG titers may not be reliable as a means to detect reactivation of latent virus. The preferred method for diagnosis is culture of the virus or detection of the antigen in infected body fluids.

IgM antibodies can be detected in adults by ELISA in primary CMV infections (93-100%). An IgM response may be reduced or absent in immunocompromised patients with active infection. The preferred method of diagnosis in these patients is culture of virus or detection of antigen. Most AIDS patients are seropositive for CMV even before HIV infection is diagnosed. Since it does not cross the placenta, detection of IgM antibody in the serum of a newborn indicates congenital infection; however, the antibody may not be present in 10-15% of infected children.

The CMV PCR assay offered at ARUP is a qualitative test. Results are reported as positive or negative for the presence of CMV viral DNA. *For Cytomegalovirus Antigenemia (0065151):* Cytomegalovirus causes substantial morbidity and mortality among immunocompromised patients. During active CMV infection, the virus disseminates in the blood, which is a significant risk factor for development of end-organ disease, such as pneumonitis, retinitis, etc. Conventional methods for CMV detection in blood, such as tube culture, are sensitive, but slow. Shell vial culture is rapid but less sensitive. Techniques that allow detection of antigens present early in viral replication, such as the antigenemia assay or amplification techniques that detect viral DNA, are both rapid and sensitive. While asymptomatic patients may develop viremia, patients with CMV disease usually have a higher viral load.

Quantification of CMV viral load in peripheral blood leukocytes or plasma has been shown to correlate with progression to disease, particularly in bone marrow transplant recipients. Measurement of viral load also provides a potential mechanism for monitoring response to therapy. More data is needed to assess thresholds of significant levels of viremia among the different immuno compromised patient groups. The CMV antigenemia assay is reported as the number of positive cells per slide (200,000 leukocytes).

Note: This test uses a kit designated by the manufacturer as "for research use, not for clinical use." The performance characteristics of this test were validated by ARUP Laboratories, Inc. The U.S. Food and Drug Administration (FDA) has not approved this test. The results are not intended to be used as the sole means for clinical diagnosis or patient management decisions. ARUP is authorized under Clinical Laboratory Improvement Amendments (CLIA) and by all states to perform high-complexity testing.

AMAS (Antimalignant Antibody and Serum test) *Clinical Significance:* AMAS is a general cancer test, independent of cell type or cancer type. It is *better in the early stages but has no value at the end stages of cancer.* It's an especially good test for otherwise healthy high-risk people in families with cancer histories to watch for early signs of cancer. Therefore, the AMAS test is the *first* test you want to use in the beginning. It works early but cannot be used late in the disease when in fact it no longer is needed. When performed within 24 hours the AMAS test is better than 99% accurate.

The AMAS test is a quantitative, immunochemical determination, giving micrograms per milliliter by spectrophotometer. There is no need for subjective measures such as interpretation of colors, shape and configuration of cells that depend on the eye of a pathologist or lab technician. Rather it measures optical density, which is then translated into micrograms per milliliter.

It is a generic test for cancers of all types and independent of specific cell types because it measures the appearance of an antigen that appears in every cancer cell in the body regardless of location. The antigen that appears in every cancer cell stimulates an immune response that produces a specific antibody to the antigen. If a cell is transformed to a malignant state regardless of its cell type it releases a substance called malignant peptide (Malignin). The body recognizes Malignin as foreign and makes an antibody against it. The AMAS test measures that specific antibody — it does NOT measure antigens.

All the other tests measure antigens (bio marker test, CEA, PSA, CA125). Tumors/cancers release antigens into the blood stream and the more cancer cells, the more antigen is released into the blood stream so antigen tests get higher as the cancer gets worse and are more and more accurate as the cancer worsens. However, since the AMAS test does *not* measure antigen but rather an antibody to the antigens — *the antibody is quickly released early on making the AMAS test better in the early stages but worthless at the end stages; because, the antibody response is wiped out in terminal or advanced cancer.* The more terminal the cancer the more obvious the clinical evidence until tests are no longer needed. It's obvious on clinical inspection of signs and symptoms and history taking.

It's an especially good test for otherwise healthy high-risk people in families with cancer histories. They should take the test periodically to watch for early signs of cancer. The AMAS test has lower false positives than the antigen tests, is elevated earlier in the disease, and returns to normal in remission. The AMAS test is Medicare approved.

For Further Information on the AMAS test have your physician contact Oncolab, Inc. m36 The Fenway Boston, MA 02215, 1-617-536-0850, 1-800-9CA-TEST (1-800-922-8378).

Note: The requisition form for the test *requires signatures of both patient and doctor* and will be returned if both signatures are not on the request form.

Overview The information provided is based on first hand clinical experience. The key points are:
- Cancer is the end result of the breakdown of the immune system.
- The tumor is a symptom *not* the disease.
- An integrated approach is often needed to solve the problem.
- Diet and food supplements boost the body's immune system and change the internal environment of the body, which prevents cancer from surviving.
- Food supplements must be tested to maximize their effectiveness.
- Cancer can be monitored by means of tumor markers.

SECTION 2 REFERENCES

References for Flax Oil

[1] "Promotion and Prevention of Tumor Growth Effects of Endotoxins, Inflammation, and Dietary Lipids", by Raymond Kearney, Ph.D., Department of Infectious Diseases, The University of Sydney, Sydney, N.S.W. 2006 Australia. International Clinical Nutrition Review, October, 1987 Vol. 7, No. 4.

[2] Roehm, "Townsend Letter for Doctors", July 1990

[3] Ed McCabe, "Oxygen Therapies"

[4] "The natural way to better health and longer life", Bullivant.

[5] Arlin J. Brown, "March of Truth On Cancer", (seventh edition). Summary of 79 nontoxic cancer treatments. Available from the Arlin J. Brown Information Centre Inc., P.O. Box 251, Fort Belvoir, Virginia, 22060. Phone: 1-703-752-9511.

Books to read

- *Flax Oil As a True Aid Against Arthritis Heart Infarction Cancer and Other Diseases* by Johanna Dr. Budwig Amazon Price: $5.56
- *The Breuss Cancer Cure: Advice for the Prevention and Natural Treatment of Cancer, Leukemia and Other Seemingly Incurable Diseases* by Rudolf Breuss Amazon Price : $11.00
- *A Cancer Therapy : Results of Fifty Cases and the Cure of Advanced Cancer by Diet Therapy : A Summary of 30 Years of Clinical Experimentation* by M. Max Gerson Amazon Price: $24.95
- *Flax Oil* by Dr Budwig */www.amazon.com/exec/obidos/ISBN=0969527217/9789-9510244-200272 www.aodr.com/Health/Alternative/Ozone_Therapy/*
- *Dr. Budwig and The Healing Power of Flaxseed* (Commercial site) *www.barleans.com/literature/flax/48-lignan-flax-oil.html*
- *Essential Fatty Acids: Are You Deficient In These Key Nutrients? www.barleans.com/literature/flax/69-efa-deficient.html*

References for Calcium

The relationship between cancer and calcium; The Calcium Factor by Dr. Carl J. RReich, M.D. and Robert R. Barefoot

References for CoQ10

[6] Dr. Atkins, monthly newsletter

[7] An introduction to CoQ10 By: Peter H. Langsjoen, M.D.

[8] web site: *faculty.washington.edu/ely/coenzq10.html*

References for Mistletoe

[1] Hulsen H, Mechelke F: In vitro effectiveness of a mistletoe preparation on cytostatic-drug-resistant human leukemia cells. Naturwissenschaften 74(3): 144-145, 1987.

[2] Janssen O, Scheffler A, Kabelitz D: In vitro effects of mistletoe extracts and mistletoe lectins: cytotoxicity towards tumor cells due to the induction of programmed cell death (apoptosis). Fortschritte Der Arzneimittelforschung. Progress in Drug Research 43(11): 1221-1227, 1993.

[3] Jung ML, Baudino S, Ribereau-Gayon G, et al.: Characterization of cytotoxic proteins from mistletoe (Viscum album L.). Cancer Letters 51(2): 103-108, 1990.

[4] Khwaja TA, Dias CB, Pentecost S: Recent studies on the anticancer activities of mistletoe (Viscum album) and its alkaloids. Oncology 43(suppl 1): 42-50, 1986.

[5] Kuttan G, Vasudevan DM, Kuttan R: Effect of a preparation from Viscum album on tumor development in vitro and in mice. Journal of Ethnopharmacology 29(1): 35-41, 1990.

[6] Ribereau-Gayon G, Jung ML, Baudino S, et al.: Effects of mistletoe (Viscum album L.) extracts on cultured tumor cells. Experientia 42(6): 594-599, 1986.

[7] Stirpe F, Sandvig K, Olsnes S, et al.: Action of viscumin, a toxic lectin from mistletoe, on cells in culture. Journal of Biological Chemistry 257(22): 13271-13277, 1982.

[8] Walzel H, Jonas L, Rosin T, et al.: Relationship between internalization kinetics and cytotoxicity of mistletoe lectin I to L1210 leukaemia cells. Folia Biologica (Praha) 36(3-4): 181-188, 1990.

[9] Schaller G, Urech K, Giannattasio M: Cytotoxicity of different viscotoxins and extracts from the European subspecies Viscum album L. Phytotherapy Research 10(6): 473-477, 1996.

[10] Bussing A, Suzart K, Bergmann J, et al.: Induction of apoptosis in human lymphocytes treated with Viscum album L. is mediated by the mistletoe lectins. Cancer Letters 99(1): 59-72, 1996.

[11] Franz H: Mistletoe lectins and their A and B chains. Oncology 43(suppl 1): 23-34, 1986.

[12] Beuth J, Ko HL, Gabius HJ, et al.: Behavior of lymphocyte subsets and expression of activation markers in response to immunotherapy with galactoside-specific lectin from mistletoe in breast cancer patients. Clinical Investigator 70(8): 658-661, 1992.

[13] Beuth J, Ko HL, Tunggal L, et al.: Immunoprotective activity of the galactoside-specific mistletoe lectin in cortisone-treated BALB/c-mice. In Vivo 8(6): 989-992, 1994.

[14] Beuth J, Ko HL, Tunggal L, et al.: Thymocyte proliferation and maturation in response to galactoside-specific mistletoe lectin-1. In Vivo 7(5): 407-410, 1993.

[15] Hajto T: Immunomodulatory effects of Iscador: a Viscum album preparation. Oncology 43(suppl 1): 51-65, 1986.

[16] Hajto T, Hostanska K, Frei K, et al.: Increased secretion of tumor necrosis factor alpha, interleukin 1, and interleukin 6 by human mononuclear cells exposed to beta-galactoside-specific lectin from clinically applied mistletoe extract. Cancer Research 50(11): 3322-3326, 1990.

[17] Hajto T, Hostanska K, Gabius HJ: Modulatory potency of the beta- galactoside-specific lectin from mistletoe extract (Iscador) on the host defense system in vivo in rabbits and patients. Cancer Research 49(17): 4803- 4808, 1989.

[18] Hajto T, Lansrein C: Natural killer and antibody-dependent cell- mediated cytotoxicity activities and large granular lymphocyte frequencies in Viscum album-treated breast cancer patients. Oncology 43(2): 93-97, 1986.

[19] Hamprecht K, Handgretinger R, Voetsch W, et al.: Mediation of human NK-activity by components in extracts of Viscum album. International Journal of Immunopharmacology 9(2): 199-209, 1987.

[20] Heiny BM, Beuth J: Mistletoe extract standardized for the galactoside-specific lectin (ML-1) induces beta-endorphin release and immunopotentiation in breast cancer patients. Anticancer Research 14: 1339-1342, 1994.

[21] Hostanska K, Hajto T, Spagnoli GC, et al.: A plant lectin derived from Viscum album induces cytokine gene expression and protein production in cultures of human peripheral blood mononuclear cells. Natural Immunity 14(5- 6): 295-304, 1995.

[22] Jurin M, Zarkovic N, Hrzenjak M, et al.: Antitumorous and immunomodulatory effects of the Viscum album L. preparation Isorel. Oncology 50(6): 393-398, 1993.

[23] Kuttan G, Kuttan R: Immunomodulatory activity of a peptide isolated from Viscum album extract (NSC 635 089). Immunological Investigations 21(4): 285-296, 1992.

[24] Kuttan G: Tumoricidal activity of mouse peritoneal macrophages treated with Viscum album extract. Immunological Investigations 22 (6-7): 431-440, 1993.

[25] Mueller EA, Hamprecht K, Anderer FA: Biochemical characterization of a component in extracts of Viscum album enhancing human NK cytotoxicity. Immunopharmacology 17(1): 11-18, 1989.

[26] Nienhaus J, Stoll M, Vester F: Thymus stimulation and cancer prophylaxis by Viscum proteins. Experientia 26(5): 523-525, 1970.

[27] Rentea R, Lyon E, Hunter R: Biologic properties of Iscador: a Viscum album preparation, I: hyperplasia of the thymic cortex and accelerated regeneration of hematopoietic cells following x-irradiation. Laboratory Investigation 44(1): 43-48, 1981.

[28] Stein G, Berg PA: Non-lectin component in a fermented extract from Viscum album L. grown on pines induces proliferation of lymphocytes from healthy and allergic individuals in vitro. European Journal of Clinical Pharmacology 47(1): 33-38, 1994.

[29] Timoshenko AV, Gabius HJ: Efficient induction of superoxide release from human neutrophils by the galactoside-specific lectin from Viscum album. Biological Chemistry Hoppe Seyler 374(4): 237-243, 1993.

[30] Timoshenko AV, Gabius HJ: Influence of the galactoside-specific lectin from Viscum album and its subunits on cell aggregation and selected intracellular parameters of rat thymocytes. Planta Medica 61(2): 130-133, 1995.

[31] Timoshenko AV, Kayser K, Drings P, et al.: Modulation of lectin-triggered superoxide release from neutrophils of tumor patients with and without chemotherapy. Anticancer Research 13(5C): 1789-1792, 1993.

[32] Chernyshov VP, Omelchenko LI, Heusser P, et al.: Immunomodulatory actions of Viscum album (Iscador) in children with recurrent respiratory disease as a result of the Chernobyl nuclear accident. Complementary Therapy and Medicine 5(3): 141-146, 1997.

[33] Beuth J, Stoffel B, Ko HL, et al.: Immunomodulating ability of galactoside-specific lectin standardized and depleted mistletoe extract. Fortschritte Der Arzneimittelforschung. Progress in Drug Research 45(11): 1240-1242, 1995.

[34] Bloksma N, Schmiermann P, de Reuver M, et al.: Stimulation of humoral and cellular immunity by Viscum preparations. Planta Medica 46(4): 221-227, 1982.

[35] Heiny BM, Albrecht V, Beuth J: Correlation of immune cell activities and beta-endorphin release in breast carcinoma patients treated with galactose-specific lectin standardized mistletoe extract. Anticancer Research 18(1B): 583-586, 1998.

[36] Lenartz D, Stoffel B, Menzel J, et al.: Immunoprotective activity of the galactoside-specific lectin from mistletoe after tumor destructive therapy in glioma patients. Anticancer Research 16(6B): 3799-3802, 1996.

[37] Stein GM, Schaller G, Pfuller U, et al.: Charaterisation of granulocyte stimulation by thionins from European mistletoe and from wheat. Biochimica et Biophysica Acta 1426(1): 80-90, 1999.

[38] Stein GM, Schaller G, Pfuller U, et al.: Thionins from Viscum album L: influence of the viscotoxins on the activation of granulocytes. Anticancer Research 19(2A): 1037-1042, 1999.

[39] Dietrich JB, Ribereau-Gayon G, Jung ML, et al.: Identity of the N-terminal sequences of the three A chains of mistletoe (Viscum album L.) lectins: homology with ricin-like plant toxins and single-chain ribosome-inhibiting proteins. Anti-Cancer Drugs 3(5): 507-511, 1992.

[40] Gabius HJ, Walzel H, Joshi SS, et al.: The immunomodulatory beta- galactoside-specific lectin from mistletoe: partial sequence analysis, cell and tissue binding, and impact on intracellular biosignalling of monocytic leukemia cells. Anticancer Research 12(3): 669-675, 1992.

[41] Holtskog R, Sandvig K, Olsnes S: Characterization of a toxic lectin in Iscador, a mistletoe preparation with alleged cancerostatic properties. Oncology 45(3): 172-179, 1988.

[42] Jaggy C, Musielski H, Urech K, et al.: Quantitative determination of lectins in mistletoe preparations. Fortschritte Der Arzneimittelforschung. Progress in Drug Research 45(8): 905-909, 1995.

[43] Olsnes S, Stirpe F, Sandvig K, et al.: Isolation and characterization of viscumin, a toxic lectin from Viscum album L. (mistletoe). Journal of Biological Chemistry 257(22): 13263-13270, 1982.

[44] Samal AB, Gabius HJ, Timoshenko AV: Galactose-specific lectin from Viscum album as a mediator of aggregation and priming of human platelets. Anticancer Research 15(2): 361-368, 1995.

[45] Schrader G, Apel K: Isolation and characterization of cDNAs encoding viscotoxins of mistletoe (Viscum album). European Journal of Biochemistry 198(3): 549-553, 1991.

[46] Sweeney EC, Palmer RA, Pfuller U: Crystallization of the ribosome inactivating protein ML1 from Viscum album (mistletoe) complexed with beta-D- galactose. Journal of Molecular Biology 234(4): 1279-1281, 1993.

[47] Timoshenko AV, Cherenkevich SN, Gabius HJ: Viscum album agglutinin-induced aggregation of blood cells and the lectin effects on neutrophil function. Biomedicine and Pharmacotherapy 49(3): 153-158, 1995.

[48] Friess H, Beger HG, Kunz J, et al.: Treatment of advanced pancreatic cancer with mistletoe: results of a pilot trial. Anticancer Research 16(2): 915-920, 1996.

[49] Khwaja TA, Varven JC, Pentecost S, et al.: Isolation of biologically active alkaloids from Korean mistletoe Viscum album, coloratum. Experientia 36(5): 599-600, 1980.

[50] Gabius HJ, Gabius S, Joshi SS, et al.: From ill-defined extracts to the immunomodulatory lectin: will there be a reason for oncological application of mistletoe? Planta Medica 60(1): 2-7, 1994.

[51] Zee-Cheng RK: Anticancer research on Loranthaceae plants. Drugs of the Future 22(5): 519-530, 1997.

52 Mistletoe: In: Murray MT: The Healing Power of Herbs. Roseville, CA: Prima Publishing, 1995: pp 253-259.

53 Kaegi E, on behalf of the Task Force on Alternative Therapies of the Canadian Breast Cancer Research Initiative: Unconventional therapies for cancer, 3: Iscador. Canadian Medical Association Journal 158(9): 1157-1159, 1998.

54 Capernaros Z: The golden bough: the case for mistletoe. European Journal of Herbal Medicine 1(1):19-24, 1994.

55 Bocci V: Mistletoe (Viscum album) lectins as cytokine inducers and immunoadjuvant in tumor therapy: a review. Journal of Biological Regulators and Homeostatic Agents 7(1): 1-6, 1993.

56 Mistletoe: In: Newall CA, Anderson LA, Phillipson JD: Herbal Medicines: A Guide for Health-Care Professionals. London, England: Pharmaceutical Press, 1996: pp 193-196.

57 Wall ME: Camptothecin and taxol: discovery to clinic. Medicinal Research Reviews 18(5): 299-314, 1998.

58 Noble RL: The discovery of vinca alkaloids – chemotherapeutic agents against cancer. Biochemistry and Cell Biology 68(12): 1344-1351, 1990.

59 Chabner BA, Horwitz SB: Plant alkaloids. In: Pinedo HM, Chabner BA, Longo DL, eds.: Cancer Chemotherapy and Biological Response Modifiers Annual 11. Amsterdam, The Netherlands: Elsevier Science Publishers, 1990: pp 74-81.

60 Kilpatrick DC: Mechanisms and assessment of lectin-mediated mitogenesis. Molecular Biotechnology 11(1): 55-65, 1999.

61 Abdullaev FI, de Mejia EG: Antitumor effect of plant lectins. Natural Toxins 5(4): 157-163, 1997.

62 Barondes SH: Lectins: their multiple endogenous cellular functions. Annual Review of Biochemistry 50: 207-231, 1981.

63 Nicolson GL: The interactions of lectins with animal cell surfaces. International Review of Cytology 39: 89-190, 1974.

64 American Cancer Society: Unproven methods of cancer management: Iscador. CA-A Cancer Journal for Clinicians 33(3): 186-188, 1983.

65 Becker H: Botany of European mistletoe (Viscum album L.). Oncology 43(suppl 1): 2-7, 1986.

66 Hauser SP: Unproven methods in oncology. European Journal of Cancer 27(12): 1549-1551, 1991.

67 Ribereau-Gayon G, Jung ML, Di Scala D, et al.: Comparison of the effects of fermented and unfermented mistletoe preparations on cultured tumor cells. Oncology 43(suppl 1): 35-41, 1986.

68 Wagner H, Jordan E, Feil B: Studies on the standardization of mistletoe preparations. Oncology 43(suppl 1): 16-22, 1986.

69 Kleijnen J, Knipschild P: Mistletoe treatment for cancer: review of controlled trials in humans. Phytomedicine 1: 255-260, 1994.

70 Fellmer KE: A clinical trial of Iscador: follow-up treatment of irradiated genital carcinomata for the prevention of recurrences. British Homeopathic Journal 57: 43-47, 1968.

71 Watkins D: A berry Christmas. Nursing Times 93(51): 28-29, 1997.

72 Samtleben R, Hajto T, Hostanska K, et al.: Mistletoe lectins as immunostimulants (chemistry, pharmacology and clinic). In: Immunomodulatory Agents from Plants, Wagner H (ed.). Basel, Switzerland: Birkhauser Verlag. 1999: 223-241.

73 Bradley GW, Clover A: Apparent response of small cell lung cancer to an extract of mistletoe and homeopathic treatment. Thorax 44(12): 1047-1048, 1989.

74 Kjaer M: Mistletoe (Iscador) therapy in stage IV renal adenocarcinoma: a phase II study in patients with measurable lung metastases. Acta Oncologica 28(4): 489-494, 1989.

75 Salzer G: Pleura carcinosis: cytomorphological findings with the mistletoe preparation Iscador and other pharmaceuticals. Oncology 43(suppl 1): 66-70, 1986.

76 Kalden VM: Klinische erfahrungen mit Viscum album bei fortgeschrittenen tumoren. Erfahrungsheilkunde 43(6): 315-321, 1994.

77 Bussing A, Lehnert A, Schink M, et al.: Effect of Viscum album L. on rapidly proliferating amniotic fluid cells: sister chromatid exchange frequency and proliferation index. Fortschritte Der Arzneimittelforschung. Progress in Drug Research 45(1): 81-83, 1995.

[78] Bussing A, Regnery A, Schweizer K: Effects of Viscum album L. on cyclophosphamide-treated peripheral blood mononuclear cells in vitro: sister chromatid exchanges and activation/proliferation marker expression. Cancer Letters 94(2): 199-205, 1995.

[79] Bussing A, Jungmann H, Suzart K, et al.: Suppression of sister chromatid exchange-inducing DNA lesions in cultured peripheral blood mononuclear cells by Viscum album L. Journal of Experimental and Clinical Cancer Research 15(2): 107-114, 1996.

[80] Bussing A, Azhari T, Ostendorp H, et al.: Viscum album L. extracts reduce sister chromatid exchanges in cultured peripheral blood mononuclear cells. European Journal of Cancer 30A(12): 1836-1841, 1994.

[81] Wiedlocha A, Sandvig K, Walzel H, et al.: Internalization and action of an immunotoxin containing mistletoe lectin A-chain. Cancer Research 51(3): 916-920, 1991.

[82] Mueller EA, Anderer A: Chemical specificity of effector cell/tumor cell bridging by a Viscum album rhamnogalacturonan enhancing cytotoxicity of human NK cells. Immunopharmacology 19(1): 69-77, 1990.

[83] Jonas L, Walzel H, Bremer H, et al.: Comparative studies on internalization of gold labelled mistletoe lectin I (MLI), its subunits, and of an immunotoxin into mouse L 1210V leukemia cells. Acta Histochemica 92(1): 46-53, 1992.

[84] Schutt C, Pfuller U, Siegl E, et al.: Selective killing of human monocytes by an immunotoxin containing partially denatured mistletoe lectin I. International Journal of Immunopharmacology 11(8): 977-980, 1989.

[85] Tonevitsky AG, Toptygin AY, Pfuller U, et al.: Immunotoxin with mistletoe lectin I A-chain and ricin A-chain directed against CD5 antigen of human T-lymphocytes: comparison of efficiency and specificity. International Journal of Immunopharmacology 13(7): 1037-1041, 1991.

[86] Yesilada E, Deliorman D, Ergun F, et al.: Effects of the Turkish subspecies of Viscum album on macrophage-derived cytokines. Journal of Ethnopharmacology 61(3): 195-200, 1998.

[87] Gawlik C, Versteeg R, Engel E, et al.: Antiproliferative effect of mistletoe-extracts in melanoma cell lines. Anticancer Research 12(6A): 364A, 1992.

[88] Kuttan G, Vasudevan DM, Kuttan R: Isolation and identification of a tumour reducing component from mistletoe extract (Iscador). Cancer Letters 41(3): 307-314, 1988.

[89] Berger M, Schmahl D: Studies on the tumor-inhibiting efficacy of Iscador in experimental animal tumors. Journal of Cancer Research and Clinical Oncology 105(3): 262-265, 1983.

[90] Kuttan G, Kuttan R: Immunological mechanism of action of the tumor reducing peptide from mistletoe extract (NSC 635089) cellular proliferation. Cancer Letters 66(2): 123-130, 1992.

[91] Kuttan G, Kuttan R: Reduction of leukopenia in mice by "Viscum album" administration during radiation and chemotherapy. Tumori 79(1): 74-76, 1993.

[92] Preisfeld A: Influence of aqueous mistletoe preparations on humoral immune parameters with emphasis on the cytotoxicity of human complement in breast cancer patients. Forschende Komplementarmedizin 4: 224-228, 1997.

[93] Kovacs E, Hajto T, Hostanska K: Improvement of DNA repair in lymphocytes of breast cancer patients treated with Viscum album extract (Iscador). European Journal of Cancer 27(12): 1672-1676, 1991.

[94] Lenartz D, Dott U, Menzel J, et al.: Survival of glioma patients after complementary treatment with galactoside-specific lectin from mistletoe. Anticancer Research 20(3B): 2073-2076, 2000.

[95] Eggermont AM, Kleeberg UR, Ruiter DJ, et al. European Organization for Research and Treatment of Cancer Melanoma Group trial experience with more than 2,000 patients, evaluating adjuvant treatment with low or intermediate doses of interferon alpha-2b. In: American Society of Clinical Oncology Educational Book, Spring 2001 (37th Annual Meeting), pp. 88-93. Note: This information is also available at *http://www.asco.org*; take the following links: ASCO Virtual Meeting Sites > 2001 ASCO Virtual Meeting > Lectures > Other Interest Areas > Adjuvant Therapy for Melanoma > Alexander M.M. Eggermont, MD, PhD, Speaker.

[96] Steuer-Vogt MK, Bonkowsky V, Ambrosch P, et al. The effect of an adjuvant mistletoe treatment programme in resected head and neck cancer patients: a randomised controlled clinical trial. European Journal of Cancer 37(1):23-31, 2001.

[97] Stettin A, Schultze JL, Stechemesser E, et al.: Anti-mistletoe lectin antibodies are produced in patients during therapy with an aqueous mistletoe extract derived from Viscum album L. and neutralize lectin-induced cytotoxicity in vitro. Klinische Wochenschrift 68(18): 896-900, 1990.

[98] Tonevitsky AG, Shamshiev AT, Prokoph'ev SA, et al.: Hybridoma cells producing antibodies against A-chain of mistletoe lectin I are resistant to this toxin. Immunology Letters 46(1-2): 5-8, 1995.

[99] Kuttan G, Vasudevan DM, Kuttan R: Presence of a receptor for the active component of Iscador in ascites fluid of tumour bearing mice. Cancer Letters 48(3): 223-227, 1989.

[100] Kannan S, Gabius HJ, Chandran GJ, et al.: Expression of galactoside-specific endogenous lectins and their ligands in human oral squamous cell carcinoma. Cancer Letters 85(1): 1-7, 1994.

[101] Hall AH, Spoerke DG, Rumack BH, et al.: Assessing mistletoe toxicity. Annals of Emergency Medicine 15(11): 1320-1323, 1986.

References for Rhodiola rosea

[4] Duhan, O.M. et al. (1999) "The antimutagenic activity of biomass extracts from the cultured cells of medicinal plants in the Ames test" Tsitol Genet Nov-Dec 33(6): 19-25

[5] Udintsev SN; et.al. (1991) "The role of humoral factors of regenerating liver in the development of experimental tumours and the effect of Rhodiola rosea extract on this process" Neoplasma: 38(3): 323-31

[6] Bocharova OA et.al. (1995) "The effect of a Rhodiola rosea extract on the incidence of recurrences of a superficial bladder cancer (experimental clinical research)" Urol Nefrol (Mosk) Mar-Apr (2): 46-7

[7] Salikhova RA et.al. (1997) "Effect of Rhodiola rosea on the yield of mutation alteration and DNA repair in bone marrow cells". Patol Fiziol Exsp Ter Oct-Dec (4): 22-4

References for Cancer Antigen 125 or CA-125

- Jacobs I and Bast RC. The CA 125 tumor-associated antigen: a review of the literature. Hum Reprod 1989; 4:1-12.
- Kang JO, et al. Enzyme-linked immunosorbent assay of CA-125 in serum of patients with endometriosis: efficacy in diagnosis. Clin Chem 1988; 34:1983-1986.
- Molina R, et al. Cancer antigen 125 in serum and ascitic fluid of patients with liver diseases. Clin Chem 1991; 37:1379-1383.

References for LASA-P

- Katopodis N and Stock CC. Improved method to determine lipid-bound sialic acid in plasma or serum. Res Commun Chem Pathol Pharmacol 1980; 30:171-180.
- Katopodis N, et al. Lipid-associated sialic acid test for the detection of human cancer. Cancer Res 1982; 42:5270-5275.
- Onistrian A and Schwartz MK. Lipid-associated sialic acid. Clin Chem News 1985; 11:14-15.

References for Cancer Antigen-Breast (CA 15-3)

- Hayes DF, et al. Clinical applications of CA 15-3. In Serological cancer markers. S Sell, ed. 1992; Totowa: Humana Press, 281-307.
- Wu JT and Erali M. Development of radioimmunoassays on microplate: application for CA-GI and CA-BR tumor markers. J Clin Lab Anal 1993; 7:341-347.

References for Cancer Antigen-G1 (CA 19-9)

- Steinberg WM, et al. Comparison of the sensitivity and specificity of the CA 19-9 and carcinoembryonic antigen assays in detecting cancer of the pancreas. Gastroenterology 1986; 90:343-349.
- Wu JT and Erali M. Development of radioimmunoassays on microplate: application for CA-GI and CA-BR tumor markers. J Clin Lab Anal 1993; 7:341-347.
- Wu JT and Christensen SE. Effect of different test designs of immunoassays on "hook effect" of CA 19-9 measurement. J Clin Lab Anal 1991; 5:228-232.

References for Cytomegalovirus (CMV)

- Achim CL, et al. Detection of cytomegalovirus in cerebrospinal fluid autopsy specimens from AIDS patients. J Infect Dis 1994; 172:623-627.

- Akrigg A, et al. The structure of the major immediate early gene of human cytomegalovirus strain AD169. Virus Research 1985; 2:107-121.
- Arribas JR, et. al. Level of cytomegalovirus (CMV) DNA in cerebrospinal fluid of subjects with AIDS and CMV infection of the central nervous system. J Infect Dis 1995; 172:527-531.
- Boeckh M and Boivin G. Quantitation of cytomegalovirus: methodologic aspects and clinical applications. J Clin Microbiol 1998; 11:533-554.
- Cinque P, et.al. Cytomegalovirus infection of the central nervous system in patients with AIDS: diagnosis by DNA amplification from cerebrospinal fluid. J Infect Dis 1992; 166:1408-1411.
- Clifford DB, et. al. Use of polymerase chain reaction to demonstrate cytomegalovirus DNA in CSF of patients with human immunodeficiency virus infection. Neurology 1993; 43:75-79.
- Drew WL. Diagnosis of cytomegalovirus infection. Rev Infect Dis 1988; 10:468-476.
- Fillet AM, et. al. Human CMV infection of the CNS and pathological examination. AIDS 1993; 7:1016-1018.
- Gozlan J, et. al. A prospective evaluation of clinical criteria and polymerase chain reaction assay of cerebrospinal fluid for the diagnosis of cytomegalovirus-related neurological diseases during AIDS. AIDS 1995; 9:253-260.
- Gozlan J, et. al. Rapid detection of cytomegalovirus DNA in cerebrospinal fluid of AIDS patients with neurologic disorders. J Infect Dis 1992; 166:1416-1421.
- Grefte JM, et. al. The lower matrix protein pp65 is the principal viral antigen present in peripheral blood leukocytes during an active cytomegalovirus infection. J Gen Virol 1992; 73:2923-2932.
- Holland NR, et al. Cytomegalovirus encephalitis in acquired immunodeficiency syndrome (AIDS). Neurology 1994; 44:507-514.
- Kalayjian RC, et al. Cytomegalovirus ventriculoencephalitis in AIDS: a syndrome with distinct clinical and pathologic features. Medicine (Baltimore) 1993; 72:67-77.
- Kim YS and Hollander H. 1993. Polyradiculopathy due to cytomegalovirus: report of two cases in which improvement occurred after prolonged therapy and review of the literature. Clin Infect Dis 1993; 17:32-37.
- Mastroianni CM, et. al. Detection of cytomegalovirus matrix protein (pt65) in leukocytes of HIV-infected patients with painful peripheral neuropathy. J Med Virology 1994; 44:172-175.
- Mazzulli T, et al. Cytomegalovirus antigenemia: clinical correlation in transplant recipients and in persons with AIDS. J Clin Microbiol 1993; 31:2824-2827.
- McCutchan JA. Clinical impact of cytomegalovirus infections of the nervous system in patients with AIDS. Clin Infect Dis 1995; 21(Suppl 2):S196-201.
- McHugh TM, et al. Comparison of six methods for the detection of antibody to cytomegalovirus. J Clin Microbiol 1985; 22:1014-1019.
- So YT and Olney RF. Acute lumbosacral polyradiculopathy in acquired immunodeficiency syndrome: experience in 23 patients. Ann Neurology 1994; 35:53-58.
- Spector SA, et. al. Molecular detection of human cytomegalovirus and determination of genotypic ganciclovir resistance in clinical specimens. Clin Infect Dis 1995; 21(Suppl 2):S170-S173.
- Van der Bij W, et al. Comparison between viremia and antigenemia for detection of cytomegalovirus in blood. J Clin Microbiol 1988; 26:2531-2535.
- Waner JL and Stewart JA. Cytomegalovirus. In *Manual of clinical laboratory* immunology, 3rd ed. NR Rose, et al, eds. 1986; Washington: Am Soc Microbiol, 504-508.
- Wolf DG and Spector SA. Diagnosis of human cytomegalovirus central nervous system disease in AIDS patients by DNA amplification from cerebrospinal fluid. J Infect Dis1992; 166:1412-1415.

"Many people would sooner die than think;
In fact, they do so."

Bertrand Russell (1872-1970)

Section 3

CHEMOTHERAPY AND ITS ADVERSE SIDE EFFECTS

CONVENTIONAL CHEMOTHERAPY

Although chemotherapy drugs attack reproducing cells, they cannot tell the difference between reproducing cells of normal tissues (that are replacing worn-out normal cells) and cancer cells. The damage to normal cells can result in side effects.

Chemotherapy involves a balance between destroying the cancer cells (in order to "cure" or control the disease) and sparing the normal cells (to lessen undesirable side effects). Chemotherapy suppresses the body's immune system. If it fails, patients are faced with three major hurtles: one, trying to regenerate the health of the immune system; two, overcoming the resistant cancer; and three, detoxification and restoring the damaged tissues. Even if chemotherapy is partially or "completely" successful, that is, the patient survives treatment, the underlying factors that caused the cancer *are still there* acting as a time bomb waiting to be triggered by an event. This latter concept is *not* being recognized by traditional medicine.

Most Common Side Effects of Chemotherapy Using chemotherapy as the primary treatment, the patient not only has to battle the cancer but also attempt repair with a damaged immune system the injuries created by the drugs. Most likely to be damaged are normal cells that divide rapidly:

- Bone marrow/blood cells
- Hair follicle cells
- Reproductive and digestive tract cells

Damage to these cells accounts for many of the side effects of chemotherapy drugs. Side effects are different for each chemotherapy drug, and they also differ based on the dosage, the route the drug takes, and how the drug affects each individual.

Bone Marrow Suppression Bone marrow is the tissue inside some bones that produces white blood cells (WBCs), red blood cells (RBCs), and blood platelets. Damage to the blood cell-producing tissues of the bone marrow is called bone marrow suppression, or myelosuppression and is one of the most common side effects of chemotherapy. Cells produced in the bone marrow tissue are growing rapidly and are sensitive to the effects of chemotherapy. Until bone marrow cells recover from this damage, there may be abnormally low numbers of WBCs, RBCs, and/or blood platelets.

While undergoing chemotherapy blood is regularly sampled, sometimes daily, so the numbers of these cells can be counted by a complete blood count (CBC). Bone marrow samples may also be taken periodically to check on the blood-forming marrow cells that develop into WBCs, RBCs, and blood platelets.

The decrease in blood cell counts does not occur immediately after chemotherapy because the drugs do not destroy the cells already in the bloodstream (which are not dividing rapidly). Instead, the drugs temporarily prevent formation of new blood cells by the bone marrow.

Each type of blood cell has a different life span:
- White blood cells average a 6-hour lifespan
- Platelets average 10 days
- Red blood cells average 120 days

As blood cells normally wear out, they are constantly replaced by the bone marrow. As these cells wear out, following chemotherapy they are not replaced, as they would be normally, and the blood cell levels begin to drop. The type and dose of the chemotherapy will influence how low the blood cell counts will drop and how long it will take for the drop to occur.

The lowest count that blood cell levels fall to is called the *nadir*. The nadir for each blood cell type will occur at different times but usually WBCs and platelets will reach their nadir within 7-14 days. RBCs live longer and will not reach their nadir for several weeks.

Knowing what the 3 types of blood cells normally do can help you understand the effects of low blood cell counts.
- White blood cells help the body fight off infections.
- Platelets help prevent bleeding by forming plugs to seal up damaged blood vessels.
- Red blood cells bring oxygen to tissues, so cells throughout the body can use that oxygen to turn certain nutrients into energy.

The side effects caused by low blood cell counts will likely be at their worst when the WBC, blood platelet, and RBC are at their nadirs or lowest value.

Low white blood cell counts The medical term for a low WBC count is *leukopenia*. Blood normally has between 4,000 and 10,000 WBCs per cubic millimeter. WBCs are divided into 2 main categories, based on how they appear under the microscope:
- *Granulocytes*, which contain granules (visible specks) in the cytoplasm of the cell, include 3 subtypes — neutrophils, eosinophils, and basophils.
- *Agranulocytes*, which do not contain granules in the cytoplasm of the cell, include 3 subtypes — lymphocytes, monocytes, and macrophages.

Granulocytes, especially neutrophils, provide an important defense against infection and are the most numerous type of WBC. *Neutropenia*, an abnormally low number of neutrophils, is the most common factor that puts people with cancer at risk for infection. The normal range of neutrophils is between 2,500 and 6,000 cells per cubic millimeter. The neutrophil count must be watched closely.

To determine how likely someone is to develop an infection, health care providers calculate a number called the *absolute neutrophil count* (ANC). Someone with an ANC of 1,000 or less is considered to be *neutropenic* and at risk of developing an infection. An ANC lower than 500 is considered severe neutropenia.

Even though a WBC count or the neutrophil count may be low, it does not mean there is an infection. These are the signs and symptoms to watch for:

- Fever
- Sore throat
- New cough or shortness of breath
- Nasal congestion
- Burning during urination
- Shaking chills
- Redness, swelling, and warmth at the site of an injury

Fever may be the first and most important sign of an infection. Call a doctor or nurse with a fever greater than or equal to 100.5 F, any signs or symptoms of infection, or shaking chills.

A health care team may take preventive care measures to reduce the risk of infection and exposure to others with infections. When WBC counts are very low, doctors often prescribe antibiotics as a preventive measure. These anti-infection drugs may be given intravenously or by mouth.

Because of the risk of infection, additional chemotherapy doses may be delayed when there is a very low white blood cell count. In some situations, doctors may prescribe growth factors to keep the WBC from falling too low so that chemotherapy can be given on schedule.

The body normally produces several growth factors (also called colony-stimulating factors) to stimulate the production of various types of blood cells. But the levels of these factors in the body are often not enough to keep up with demands during chemotherapy. Scientists have recently learned how to produce these growth factors in the laboratory so they are now available as drugs.

The two growth factors that stimulate production of white blood cells are granulocyte-macrophage colony-stimulating factor (GM-CSF, sargramostim, Leukine) and granulocyte colony-stimulating factor (G-CSF, filgrastim, Neupogen). These drugs are often given daily, starting the day after chemotherapy, for up to 2 weeks. A newer, longer lasting form of

G-CSF (pegfilgrastim, Neulasta) is now available and may need to be given only once each chemotherapy cycle.

These drugs help bone marrow recover more quickly and reduce the risk of serious infection. They are given intravenously (IV) or as injections under the skin (SQ).

Nurses give the injections in the hospital or at the doctor's office, but the patient or your family members can learn how to give these injections at home.

Low red blood cell counts Not having enough red blood cells is called *anemia*. Doctors use 2 measurements to determine if there are enough RBCs.

- The red pigment in RBCs that carries oxygen is *hemoglobin*. If there are not enough RBCs, the blood hemoglobin concentration will be less than its usual range of 12 to 16 grams per deciliter (g/dL) in women or 14 to 18 g/dL in men.

- Hematocrit is the percentage of total blood volume occupied by red blood cells. Its normal range is between 37% and 52%. Levels are normally higher for men than for women.

    Anemia may produce the following symptoms:

    - Fatigue
    - Dizziness
    - Headaches
    - Irritability
    - Shortness of breath
    - An increase in heart rate or rate of breathing or both

    Anemia caused by chemotherapy is usually temporary. But bleeding caused by surgery or the cancer (a common occurrence with colorectal cancers, for example) can make anemia even worse.

Blood transfusions may be needed until the bone marrow is healthy enough to replace worn-out RBCs. Because blood transfusions have some risks, doctors use this procedure only if they see significant signs and symptoms, such as shortness of breath and/or very low RBC counts. Other factors will also affect this decision. For example, people with heart or lung diseases are more sensitive to anemia. A newer option for treating anemia caused by chemotherapy is erythropoietin (EPO, Procrit, Epogen). This naturally occurring growth factor stimulates RBC production by bone marrow cells. It can relieve symptoms of anemia and reduce the need for blood transfusions. Erythropoietin is generally given 3 times per week by injection under the skin (SQ) until the hemoglobin level increases to 12 g/dL. A newer, longer lasting form, known as darbepoietin (Aranesp), may reduce the number of injections to every 1 to 2 weeks.

Low platelet counts The normal range for platelet counts is between 150,000 and 450,000 per cubic millimeter. The medical term for a low platelet count is *thrombocytopenia*.

These are the signs of a low platlet count:

- Bruise easily
- Bleed longer than usual after minor cuts or scrapes
- Bleeding gums or nose bleeds
- Develop ecchymoses (large bruises) and petechiae (multiple small bruises)
- Serious internal bleeding if the platelet count is very low

Although low platelet counts resulting from chemotherapy are temporary, they can cause serious blood loss from injury or bleeding that can damage internal organs.

Sometimes a low platelet count will delay necessary surgery because of concern for blood loss. If platelet counts are very low (below 10,000) or if a person with moderately low counts has greater than normal bleeding or bruising, platelet transfusions may be given. *A little known fact to most physicians is that sesame oil contains a factor T, which if given daily will raise platelet levels in three to six weeks.*

Transfused platelets last only a few days, and some people who have received many platelet transfusions can develop an immune reaction that destroys donor platelets. A platelet growth factor called oprelvekin (Neumega) can be given to people with severe thrombocytopenia. This decreases their need for platelet transfusions and can stop increased bleeding. It is given under the skin every day.

Hematopoietic stem cell transplantation Hematopoietic stem cell transplantation (HSCT) is the term now used to include bone marrow transplantation (BMT) and peripheral blood stem cell transplantation (PBSCT). These transplants permit the use of especially high doses of chemotherapy and/or total body irradiation (TBI) to kill the cancer cells. In the process of wiping out the cancer, normal hematopoietic (blood forming) stem cells in the bone marrow are also killed. Therefore, stem cells are removed from the blood or bone marrow before treatment and are given back once it is completed. Another option is to receive stem cells from another person (a donor).

Hair Loss Chemotherapy affects the rapidly growing cells of hair follicles. Hair may become brittle and break off at the surface of the scalp, or it may simply fall out from the hair follicle.

Basic facts about hair loss:

- Hair loss can be very individual. Some people may have complete loss of hair while others may see just a thinning. Loss of eyebrows, eyelashes, pubic hair, and body hair is usually less severe because, the growth is less active in these hair follicles than in the scalp.
- Hair loss depends on the choice of drugs, their doses, and the length of treatment.
- If hair is going to be affected, it may happen 2 to 3 weeks after treatment begins.
- Hair loss from chemotherapy is almost always temporary.

- Hair may start to grow again near the end of treatment or after the treatment is completed.
- When hair grows back, its color or texture may be different.
- Unlike some other side effects of chemotherapy, hair loss is never life threatening. But it may have a substantial impact on quality of life. Hair loss may cause depression, loss of self-confidence, and grief.

Appetite Loss and Weight Loss *Anorexia* is a decrease in or complete loss of appetite. Most chemotherapy medications cause some degree of anorexia. Anorexia may be mild, or it may lead to *cachexia,* a form of malnutrition. Loss of appetite, as well as weight loss, may result directly from effects of the cancer on the body's metabolism.

Proper nutrition helps strengthen the body to fight the disease and cope with treatment. Decreased appetite is generally temporary and returns when chemotherapy is finished. It may take several weeks after chemotherapy is finished for the appetite to recover. Some chemotherapy may cause more severe loss of appetite.

If the patient experiences anorexia or cachexia, medications or natural B-complex vitamins can be prescribed to deal with these conditions.

Taste Changes Cancer treatments and the cancer itself can change the way some food tastes. Taste changes can contribute to anorexia and malnutrition. With taste changes caused by chemotherapy, the following may occur:

- Either a dislike for or an increased desire for sweet foods
- Dislike of foods with bitter tastes
- Dislike for tomatoes and tomato products
- Dislike for beef or pork
- Constant metallic or medicinal taste in the mouth

These changes occur because chemotherapy drugs can change the taste receptor cells in the mouth that signal what flavor are tasted. Changes in taste and smell may continue as long as chemotherapy treatments continue, or longer. Several weeks after chemotherapy has ended, taste and smell sensations usually (but not always) return to normal.

Stomatitis and Esophagitis *Stomatitis* is an inflammation and sores within the mouth that may result from chemotherapy. Similar changes in the throat or the esophagus (the tube that leads from the throat to the stomach) are called *pharyngitis* and *esophagitis.* The term *mucositis* refers to inflammation of the lining layer of the mouth, throat, and esophagus.

The first signs of mouth sores occur when the lining of the mouth appears pale and dry. Later, the mouth, gums, and throat may feel sore and become red and inflamed. The tongue may be "coated" and swollen, leading to difficulty swallowing, eating, or talking.

Stomatitis, pharyngitis, and esophagitis can lead to bleeding, painful ulceration, and infection.

Mouth, throat, and esophagus sores are temporary and usually develop 5 to 14 days after chemotherapy. They will heal completely once chemotherapy is finished.

Nausea and Vomiting Although there are new medications to both prevent and treat nausea and vomiting, it is a possible side effect of chemotherapy. Chemotherapy agents cause nausea and vomiting for a variety of reasons. They irritate the lining of the stomach and duodenum (the first section of the small intestine). This stimulates certain nerves that lead to the vomiting center in the brain.

- *Nausea* is an unpleasant wavelike sensation in the stomach and back of throat. Sweating, light-headedness, dizziness, and weakness can accompany it. It can lead to retching, vomiting, or both.
- *Retching* is a rhythmic movement of the diaphragm and stomach muscles that are controlled by the vomiting center.
- *Vomiting* is a process controlled by the vomiting center that causes the contents of the stomach to be forced out through the mouth.

Vomiting can occur at various times. It can be *acute*, occurring within minutes to hours after chemotherapy, or *delayed*, developing or continuing for 24 hours after chemotherapy and sometimes lasting for days. *Anticipatory vomiting* occurs when there has been a bad experience with nausea and vomiting in the past that was not treated. As a result, nausea and vomiting develop when the patient is placed in the same situation (for example, before receiving the next chemotherapy treatments).

Although it is not possible to predict the onset, severity, or duration of nausea and vomiting, certain chemotherapy medications are more likely to cause nausea and vomiting. *Some examples of these are:*

- Cisplatin
- Dacarbazine
- Mechlorethamine
- Daunorubicin
- Streptozocin
- Cytarabine (high doses)
- Doxorubicin
- Carmustine
- Cyclophosphamide
- Ifosfamide
- Procarbazine
- Lomustine
- Dactinomycin

- Plicamycin
- Methotrexate (high doses)
- Carboplatin

Factors that may affect the amount and severity of nausea and vomiting:
- Prior experiences with motion sickness
- Previous bad experiences with nausea and vomiting
- Being young
- Heavy alcohol intake
- Being a woman of menstrual age (at greatest risk for severe and long-lasting nausea and vomiting)

Many drugs are used alone or in combination to prevent or decrease nausea and vomiting. They include the following:
- Lorazepam
- Prochlorperazine
- Promethazine
- Metoclopramide
- Dexamethasone
- Ondansetron
- Granisetron

The key to effective control is to prevent nausea and vomiting before it occurs. Consideration may also be given to non-drug methods to help with nausea and vomiting, such as:
- Ginger in tablets or in natural ginger ale
- Taking the anti-oxidant Glutathione before, during and after treatment
- Coffee enemas to clean the liver and reduce chemotherapy metabolites
- Relaxation exercises
- Guided imagery
- Soothing music
- Drinking eight to ten (8-10) glasses of water daily

Constipation Constipation is the passage (usually with discomfort) of infrequent, hard, dry stool. Excessive straining, bloating, increased gas, cramping, or pain may also accompany constipation. Constipation affects about half of people with cancer and about 3 out of 4 of those with advanced disease.

Risk factors for developing constipation include:

- Taking opioid pain medications
- Decreased physical activity
- Poor diet
- Decreased fluid intake and dehydration
- Bed rest
- Depression
- Certain chemotherapy agents (such as vincristine and vinblastine)
- Underactive thyroid

If constipation develops, a doctor may have to determine the cause, then take appropriate measures to treat the problem.

Diarrhea Diarrhea is the passage of loose or watery stools three or more times a day with or without discomfort. Diarrhea may also be accompanied by gas, cramping, and bloating. Diarrhea occurs in about three out of four people who receive chemotherapy because of the damage to the rapidly dividing cells in the digestive (gastrointestinal) tract.

Factors affecting diarrhea during chemotherapy:

- Receiving drugs that cause diarrhea (examples include irinotecan, 5-fluorouracil, methotrexate, docetaxel, and actinomycin-D)
- The drug dose
- Length of treatment
- Having a stomach tumor
- Receiving both radiation and chemotherapy
- Being lactose intolerant (can't drink milk, for example)

Diarrhea can be serious and become life threatening if dehydration, malnutrition, and electrolyte imbalances occur. It is important to report any diarrhea to a doctor or nurse. Keep a record of the number of times, the amount, and the appearance of the diarrhea for the doctor.

Fatigue Fatigue is a common side effect of cancer and chemotherapy. Fatigue caused by chemotherapy may cause:

- Weariness
- Weakness
- Lack of energy
- Decreased ability for physical and mental work
- Difficulty thinking
- Forgetfulness
- Inability to concentrate

The fatigue a person with cancer feels is different from the fatigue of everyday life. It is unrelated to activity and may not be resolved with rest or sleep. Fatigue can be prolonged and affect quality of life. Utilizing a good nutritional program, as discussed later in this book, to support the adrenal glands, thyroid, liver and taking Optygen™ to increase oxygenation of tissues will greatly reduce the fatigue factor.

Heart Damage Certain chemotherapy drugs can damage the heart. The most common one's are daunorubicin and doxorubicin (Adriamycin). This occurs in about 1 in 10 people who receive these drugs and usually involves changes to the heart muscles. Heart damage caused by chemotherapy may bring on these symptoms:

- Puffiness or swelling in the hands and feet
- Shortness of breath
- Dizziness
- Erratic heartbeats
- Dry cough

Heart damage from a second round of mid-chest radiation may occur if there are existing heart problems like uncontrolled high blood pressure or if the patient smokes.

Before chemotherapy starts, heart function will be checked to make sure that there are no major problems. During the treatments, heart function will be checked to ensure that no changes have occurred. Tests such as an electrocardiogram (ECG), an echocardiogram, or a MUGA scan are done to check for any changes in heart function. With a MUGA scan, a radioactive substance is traced through the heart with a special scanner.

If problems develop, the chemotherapy drug will be stopped to prevent further permanent damage. Notify a doctor or nurse if there are changes in heart rhythm, weight gain, or fluid retention.

Nervous System Changes Some chemotherapy drugs can cause direct or indirect changes in the central nervous system (brain and spinal cord), the cranial nerves, or peripheral nerves. The cranial nerves are connected directly to the brain and are important for movement and touch sensation of the head, face, and neck. Cranial nerves are also important for vision, hearing, taste, and smell. Peripheral nerves lead to and from the rest of the body and are important in movement, touch sensation, and regulating activities of some internal organs.

Side effects that are the result of nerve damage caused by chemotherapy can occur soon after chemotherapy or years later. *Changes in the central nervous system could produce these symptoms:*

- Stiff neck
- Headache
- Nausea and vomiting

- Lethargy or sleepiness
- Fever
- Confusion
- Depression
- Seizures

Peripheral nervous system changes usually affect the hands and feet and can include:
- Numbness
- Tingling
- Decreased sensation

The patient may feel clumsy and have difficulty in daily activities such as opening jars or squeezing toothpaste tubes.

One of the most commonly used drugs that cause peripheral nerve damage is vincristine. If the chemotherapy is decreased or stopped, the symptoms will usually decrease or disappear. However, there are times when the damage may be permanent.

Damage to the cranial nerves may cause these symptoms:
- Visual difficulties (such as blurred vision or double vision)
- Increased sensitivity to odors
- Hearing loss or ringing in the ears
- Dry mouth

Cognitive Changes Recent research has shown that chemotherapy can also affect the way the brain functions many years after treatment. This occurs in a small number of patients and is often worse with larger doses of chemotherapy agents. Some of the brain's activities that are affected are concentration, memory, comprehension (understanding), and reasoning.

The changes that were discovered in patients are subtle, but the one's who have problems notice the differences in their thinking. Patients who have had chemotherapy and have cognitive impairment call this experience "chemo-brain" or "chemo-fog". Researchers are not sure exactly why chemotherapy affects the brain in this way or exactly how much chemotherapy (or in what combinations) it takes to cause a problem.

Researchers are currently studying the problem to get more information to help prevent and treat cognitive impairment of chemotherapy patients. There are programs that can help improve memory and problem-solving abilities. Simply being aware that problems with thinking can occur may help patients and their family members feel less isolated and alone.

Lung Damage It is possible for some chemotherapy drugs, such as bleomycin, to cause irreversible damage to the lungs. The likelihood of this occurring is increased if there is radiation to the chest in addition to chemotherapy. Age seems to be an important factor in the development of lung damage. For example, people over 70 years old have three times the risk of developing lung problems from the drug bleomycin.

Lung damage may cause symptoms such as shortness of breath, a nonproductive (dry) cough, and possibly fever. If the chemotherapy drug is stopped early enough, the lung tissue can regenerate. Because early lung changes may not show up on a chest x-ray, the lungs can be assessed through pulmonary function tests and arterial blood gas tests.

Reproduction and Sexuality Reproductive and sexual problems can occur after chemotherapy. Which, if any, reproductive problems develop depends on age, dose, and duration of the chemotherapy, and the chemotherapy.

Sexual changes men may experience:

- Most men on chemotherapy still have normal erections. A few, however, may develop problems.
- Erections and sexual desire often decrease just after a course of chemotherapy but usually recover in a week or two. A few chemotherapy drugs, for example, cisplatin or vincristine, can permanently damage parts of the nervous system. Although it is not yet proven, these drugs may interfere with the nerves that control erection.
- Chemotherapy can sometimes affect sexual desire and erections by slowing down the production of testosterone. Some of the medications used to prevent nausea during chemotherapy can also upset a man's hormonal balance, but hormone levels should return to normal after treatments have ended.
- Many chemotherapy drugs can affect sperm and the parts of the body that produce them. Some of these effects may be permanent. Freezing sperm prior to chemotherapy is one option for men who wish to father children after treatment. Although it is possible to conceive during chemotherapy, the toxicity of some drugs may cause birth defects. Therefore, couples should take precautions and use a reliable type of birth control if they are sexually active.
- Chemotherapy may suppress the immune system. Genital herpes or genital wart infections may flare-up during chemotherapy.

Sexual changes women may experience:

- Many chemotherapy drugs can either temporarily or permanently damage a woman's ovaries, reducing their output of hormones. This affects a woman's fertility and libido. Ovarian function is less likely to return in women over age 30 and they are more likely to go into menopause.
- Even though menstrual cycles may be disrupted or stopped with chemotherapy, it may still be possible to become pregnant, if some form of birth control is not used.
- Symptoms of early menopause include hot flashes, vaginal dryness and tightness during

intercourse, and irregular or no menstrual periods. As the lining of the vagina thins, light spotting of blood after intercourse becomes common.

- Some chemotherapy drugs irritate all mucous membranes in the body. This includes the lining of the vagina, which often becomes dry and inflamed.

- Vaginal infections are common during chemotherapy, particularly in women taking steroids or the powerful antibiotics used to prevent bacterial infections. Yeast cells are a natural part of the vagina's cleansing system. If too many grow, however, there may be itching inside the vagina. There may also be whitish discharge that often looks like cottage cheese. Yeast infections inflame the lining of the vagina so that intercourse burns. Yeast infections can often be prevented by not wearing pantyhose, nylon panties, and tight pants. Loose clothing and cotton panties let the vagina breathe. The doctor may also prescribe a vaginal cream or suppository to reduce yeast cells or other organisms that grow in the vagina.

- If present before, genital herpes or genital wart infections may flare-up during chemotherapy. It is especially important to have a vaginal infection treated before taking chemotherapy. The body's immune system is not as strong because of the treatment, and any infection is a greater problem.

- Chemotherapy is often given through an IV tube into the bloodstream. However, new ways have been developed to bring drugs directly to a tumor. For cancer of the bladder, for example, a liquid is placed directly into the bladder through a catheter in the urethra. Such a treatment has only a minor effect on a woman's sex life. There may be some pain during intercourse soon after the treatment. This is because the bladder and urethra are still irritated.

- For tumors in the pelvis, chemotherapy may be given by pelvic infusion. The drugs are put into the arteries that feed the tumor and give an extra strong dose to the genital area. Because this method is fairly new, doctors do not yet know the long-term effects on a woman's sex life. The immediate side effects are most likely similar to those of IV chemotherapy.

- For cancer of the ovaries or colon, the cavity around the intestines is filled with drugs in liquid form. This way of giving chemotherapy is called the intraperitoneal "belly bath." Because the chemotherapy causes the area to swell temporarily, a woman looks as if she is pregnant, which may cause her more emotional distress.

Liver Damage The liver is the organ that metabolizes, or breaks down, most of the chemotherapy drugs that enter the body. Unfortunately, some drugs can cause liver damage, including methotrexate, cytarabine (ara-C), high-dose cisplatin, high-dose cyclophosphamide, vincristine, vinblastine, and doxorubicin (Adriamycin). Most often the damage is temporary, and the liver recovers a few weeks after the drug is stopped.

Signs of liver damage:

- A yellowing of the skin and the whites of the eyes (jaundice)
- Fatigue
- Pain under the lower part of the right ribs or right upper abdomen
- Blood tests will be necessary to watch for possible liver damage. People who are older or who have hepatitis may be more likely to develop liver damage.

Kidney and Urinary System Damage Many of the breakdown products of chemotherapy drugs are excreted through the kidneys. These drug byproducts can damage the kidneys, ureters, and bladder. A history of kidney problems may place the patient at a higher risk for kidney damage. Certain chemotherapy drugs such as cisplatin, high-dose methotrexate, ifosfamide, and streptozocin are more likely to cause kidney and urinary damage than other medications.

Signs of possible kidney problems:

- Headache
- Pain in the lower back
- Fatigue
- Weakness
- Nausea
- Vomiting
- Increased blood pressure
- Increased rate of breathing
- Change in pattern of urination
- Change in color of urine
- Urgent need to urinate
- Swelling or puffiness of the body

   Blood tests to measure kidney function are done regularly to watch for any changes.

LONG-TERM SIDE EFFECTS OF CHEMOTHERAPY

For many people with cancer, chemotherapy is the best option for controlling their disease. However, there may be long-term side effects related to chemotherapy treatments.

   Side effects related to specific chemotherapy drugs can continue after the treatment is completed. These effects can progress and become chronic, or new side effects may occur. Long-term side effects depend on the specific drugs received and whether other treatments such as radiation therapy were administered.

- *Permanent organ damage:* Certain chemotherapy drugs may permanently damage the body's organs. If the damage is detected during treatment, the drug will be stopped. However, some of the side effects may remain. Damage to some organs and systems, such as the reproductive system, may not show up until after chemotherapy is finished.

- *Delayed development in children:* When young children receive chemotherapy, it may affect their growth and their ability to learn. Several factors affect long-term side effects, including the age of the child, the specific drugs, the dosage and length of treatment, and if chemotherapy is used along with other types of treatment such as radiation.

- *Nerve damage:* Nervous system changes can develop months or years after treatment. Signs of nerve damage may include hearing loss or tinnitus (ringing in the ears), sensations in the hands and feet, personality changes, sleepiness, impaired memory, shortened attention span, and seizures.

- *Blood in the urine:* Hemorrhagic cystitis (blood in the urine), a side effect of cyclophosphamide and ifosfamide, can continue for some time after the drug is stopped, and symptoms may become worse.

- *Another cancer:* Development of a second cancer is a great concern for cancer survivors. Secondary cancers can include Hodgkin disease and non-Hodgkin lymphoma (also called Hodgkin's disease and non-Hodgkin's lymphoma), leukemias, and some solid tumors. Follow-up care after all treatment is finished is an essential component of cancer care for all cancer survivors.

Logic would dictate that an active program focusing on restoring the immune system, detoxifying heavy metals and chemicals and supplying vital foods and nutrients should be routine for all cancer patients. Taking a passive role with invasive monitoring methods (x-rays, CT scans, mammograms, etc.) is a prescription for relapse.

"A wise man should consider that health is the greatest of human blessings, and learn how by his own thought to derive benefit from his illness."

Hippocrates (460 BC-377 BC)

Section 4

4

DETOXIFICATION

The detoxification process is an essential part of basic cancer therapy and must be the first priority in beginning treatment. Detoxification is generally ignored in research and clinical practice. Despite all efforts, even today many patients are lost who respond well to the cancer treatment but who are not able to excrete the products of tumor lysis or breakdown. Without sufficient detoxification neither immunotherapy nor chemotherapy will achieve long-term results.

Before any therapy is initiated, the body must be cleansed. The key factor with cancer is removing the poisons as fast as possible to permit the organs of detoxification (liver, kidneys, intestines, lymphatics and skin) to handle the toxins that will be liberated as the cancer breaks down. It is absolutely imperative that the patient carefully follows the detoxification process even after the supplements begin stimulating the release of wastes and debris. It is also extremely vital that detox in the form of coffee enemas be performed after each Rife, IPT, Oxidative and even chemotherapy. These treatments are designed to rapidly destroy cancer cells. The liberated poisonous wastes *must* be removed as quickly as possible. Doctor Kelly poignantly drives home the significance of this concept in his statement, "a person very rarely dies of cancer. It is always starvation and toxicity. These waste products accumulate and gradually overburden the body. Most persons then die of toxemia."

COFFEE ENEMAS

The coffee enema is specifically designed to stimulate the liver to dump its toxic wastes. Caffeinated organic coffee facilitates the process by dilating the portal vein leading to the liver. The coffee enema also has beneficial effects in cleaning the colon. Coffee is an excellent solvent for encrusted waste accumulated along the walls of the colon. The caffeine also directly stimulates peristaltic waves by rhythmically contracting the smooth muscles of the intestinal walls more powerfully to loosen deposits. Occasionally visible debris appears as hard, black material and "ropes" of mucus. Gradually, as the protein metabolism of the body improves, the muscle tone of the bowel becomes normal and thorough evacuation is possible without the aid of the enema.

Understanding the function and benefits of coffee enemas helps break down psychological barriers against them. Ignorance and possibly childhood fears of the enema, as well as misunderstanding the proper procedure for taking it bring about such aversion. Properly administered, the enema relieves distress, creates a sense of well-being and a feeling of cleanliness never before experienced. The proper removal of toxins and debris from the colon is absolutely essential in all conditions of disease and ill health.

Since the body goes through a detoxification process normally during the sleeping hours, it is most desirable to take the coffee enema early in the evening. This helps take the burden off the liver during the process. In active cancer cases or severe illnesses, enemas should be given twice a day (upon arising and 3:00pm or early evening). The more toxic the patient the quicker one must remove the poisons. Enemas using coffee in the evening may interfere with sound sleep. If this presents a problem, use a weaker solution to permit sleep.

How To Make A Coffee Enema

- Purchase caffeinated organic coffee beans (blonde blend and enema equipment available from *www.sawilsons.com*). Use 2 to 3 tablespoons of freshly ground beans per pint and dilute to one quart. Prepare one pint of coffee using only high quality spring, distilled or reverse osmosis water in a ceramic, glass or stainless steel saucepan with a lid. Boil lightly for three minutes, and then simmer for 17 minutes. *Strain, do not filter.* Using standard white paper filters will result in the chlorinated bleaching agent being absorbed into the coffee. *Do not use chlorinated/fluorinated tap water!* Allow coffee to cool to room temperature before use. Retain solution for 12 to15 minutes.
- If the coffee enema causes jitters, shakes, nervousness, nausea, or light-headedness, the coffee solution is too strong. The amount of coffee can be adjusted from 1 teaspoon to 4 tablespoons per quart of water as tolerance level permits.
- Periodically patients (some adults and frequently children) may encounter difficulty retaining one quart. Under such circumstances use only a pint (2 cups) of enema solution at a time. If this is the case, take 2 enemas, one right after the other, and hold each for 12 to 15 minutes as directed.

How To Take A Coffee Enema Attempt a normal bowel movement. The enema is much more effective if the colon has been evacuated. One should not become disturbed, however, if there are no regular bowel movements, or very few, during the detox program. In many cases, not enough bulk collects to instigate a normal bowel movement. When no normal bowel movements are forthcoming, the enema has cleaned the colon adequately.

With constipation the patient should increase water consumption, take three tablets of Cataplex® B (increases tone of the smooth muscle of the colon) and two wafers of Lactic Acid Yeast (acidifies the colon to promote growth of healthy bacteria) with each meal (both supplements are from Standard Process Labs; available from ICRN, Inc. 1-800-272-2323); increase bulk by adding either ground flax seeds or purchase Psyllium Husks at the health food store; take 2 tablespoons with each meal. Also make sure a quality probiotic (Natren®'s Healthy Trinity® or Bio-K Plus® 1-800-593-2465) is taken to replace the healthy bacteria in the colon. These approaches are quite helpful in forming stools and creating more normal bowel movements for those who take daily enemas.

- Standard enema bags are available at most pharmacies. On average the enema bag lasts about 2 years.
- The enema tip on the end of the hose is not adequate to give a "high enema." You may have to visit a medical supply store to obtain a plastic rectal catheter or tube about 18 inches long.
- Next, allow the coffee to flow to the end of the colon tube, thus eliminating trapped air.
- The colon tube should be lubricated with olive oil, Vitamin E oil or any other lubricant that is not a petroleum based product and doesn't contain additives or chemicals.
- If possible insert the tube 12 to 20 inches into the rectum. This should be done slowly, in a rotating motion that helps to keep the tube from "kinking up" inside the colon.
- The enema bag should not be over 36 inches higher than the rectum. If it is placed too high, the coffee runs into the colon too fast and under too much pressure, causing discomfort. The flow regulating plastic device provided with most units will regulate the coffee flow.
- The easiest position for most people is to lie on the left side until the solution is out of the bag. The enema should never be taken while sitting on the toilet or standing.
- Some people's colons have kinks or turns in them that may prevent the tube from being inserted even 18 inches. Often, if a little bit of the solution is allowed to flow into the colon as the tube is being inserted, one may comfortably get past these kinks.
- If a kink in the colon bends the tube too much and stops the flow of liquid, then insert the tube only as far as it will go while still allowing the liquid to flow freely.
- Sometimes, if one hits a kink that stops the flow of the liquid completely, the tube can be pulled out slowly just to the point where the solution is felt flowing again. Frequently, the tube can be pushed back in, past the turn that previously stopped the liquid.
- Because of the shapes and formations of some people's colons, or of course if a child is

being given the enema, it will be possible to insert the tube only a few inches. Occasionally, this is a permanent situation. Often, however, as the colon is cleaned and healed, the tube can eventually be inserted further. The tube should *never* be forced when discomfort occurs.

- After the flow of the solution is complete, remove the colon tube, although it isn't necessary. Regardless of the position used up to this point, one should now lie on the left side for at least 5 minutes, then on the back for another 5 minutes, then on the right side for at least 5 minutes.
- Those who have excessive gas may leave the tube in the colon with the hose clamp open. This allows gas to escape through the enema container. Frequently, the coffee will go in and out of the enema bag or bucket until the gas is removed/dissipated.
- After the enema is retained for 12 to 15 minutes or longer, it may be expelled.
- If there is a lot of gas and it is difficult to retain the enema, try putting 2 tablespoons of Bulgaricum into the coffee solution. The *Lactobacillus bulgaricus* helps detoxifies the unhealthy bacteria to reduce gas formation.
- If a sudden gas bubble forms causing an urge to expel the solution, breathe very fast through the nose using your abdominal muscles like a bellows. This usually helps the colon wall break up the gas bubble.
- If a little coffee leaks out, place an old towel under the buttocks.

HERBAL C*

Herbal C is a proprietary blend of sixteen different herbs that work to cleanse the blood, liver, kidneys, intestines and are known to be effective against cancer. The herbal blend is made into a concentrate or stock solution. The recommended dosage is two ounces of the stock solution and two ounces of spring water. The mixture is taken three times a day between meals. Caution is advised. The more toxic the patient the greater the chances these symptoms might appear: flu-like feeling, sweating, dizziness, diarrhea and/or constipation, bad breath, rashes, foul smelling stools and headaches. Not all toxic patients will experience all these symptoms. It is best to start off slowly, that is, take one dose per day for three days then increase to two doses per day for another three days then maintain a schedule of three doses per day thereafter.

This product is only available from ICNR, Inc. Cost $25 for a one-month supply. Check the web site: *www.icnr.com* or call 1-800-272-2323.

PRIMAL DEFENSE™*

Primal Defense™ is a natural whole food probiotic blend of HSOs™ (Homeostatic Soil Organisms). SBOs (Soil Based Organisms) are designed to optimize the health of the human digestive tract and immune system. Primal Defense™ is produced using the Poten-Zyme™ process and the Microflora Delivery System™. Primal Defense™ contains the same nutrients that have been used for thousands of years by some of the healthiest and longest living people in the world.

Beneficial soil and plant based microbes used to be ingested as part of food grown in rich, unpolluted soil. However, for the last 50 years we have been sterilizing our soil with pesticides and herbicides, destroying most bacteria both bad and good. Our modern lifestyle, which includes antibiotic drug use, chlorinated water, chemical ingestion, pollution and poor diet, is responsible for eradicating much of the beneficial bacteria in our bodies. A lack of beneficial microbes often results in poor intestinal and immune system health, contributing to a wide range of symptoms and illnesses.

The following symptoms may result from a lack of probiotics:

- Gas, Bloating and Indigestion
- Diarrhea and/or Constipation
- Bad Breath and Body Odor
- Candida Yeast Infections
- Chronic Fatigue and Fibromyalgia
- Parasites
- IBS (Irritable Bowel Syndrome)
- Skin problems such as Acne, Eczema and Psoriasis
- Delayed development in children
- High Cholesterol Levels
- Frequent Colds and Flu

Primal Defense (Homeostatic Soil Organisms) for Parasites and Candida From the book *Beyond Probiotics* by Ann Louise Gittleman:

"In the human gastrointestinal tract there are hundreds of microscopic life forms that live in a symbiotic relationship with one another. When the immune system breaks down, the body is left wide open for invasion of pathogenic organisms such as Candida (yeast) and parasites. When taken on a daily basis, the Primal Defense™ HSO's set up a protective grid in the body and stimulate the immune system to ward off against all forms of bacteria, yeast, fungi and parasites. When the Primal Defense™ HSO's colonize in the gastrointestinal tract there is simply no place for the pathogenic organisms to live. Primal Defense™ HSO's change the intestinal environment and can prevent the body from infestation of these dangerous organisms. Without Primal Defense™ HSO's, parasites and Candida are free to wreak havoc in the digestive tracts of susceptible individuals.

Parasitic Infection (Parasites) Recent medical research suggest that 3 out of 5 Americans will be infected by parasites, at some point in their lives! Often going undetected, they live off of our bodies and reproduce rapidly. Parasites can rob the body of essential nutrients and can lead to serious illness or even death. (See the book *Guess What Came To Dinner* by Ann Louise Gittleman, Avery Publications 1993, for more information on parasites.)

Candidiasis (Candida) Everyone has Candida, a form of yeast that is normally found in the human digestive tract, the vagina, and on the skin. In healthy individuals with strong, functioning immune systems, it is harmless and kept in check by the beneficial bacteria occupying the same space. When the balance of intestinal bacteria is altered and the immune system becomes compromised, Candida begins to proliferate, infecting organs and tissues of the body. The Candida becomes pathogenic, transforming from a simple benign yeast into an aggressive fungus that can severely compromise one's health."

What are HSOs™ (Homeostatic Soil Organisms)? The main component in Primal Defense™ is the HSOs™, which have been used for over 22 years by thousands of health practitioners. The naturally occurring colony arrays of probiotics are non-mutated from the original cultures found in unpolluted soil and plants and are now cultured in U.S. laboratories using the discoverer's proprietary methods. The HSOs™ are in a substrate of nutrient rich superfoods providing vitamins, minerals, trace elements, enzymes and proteins. The probiotics are then made dormant using the Microflora Delivery System™, which protects the probiotics and delivers them directly to the GI tract where they multiply and flourish.

How does HSOs™ Work? Impervious to stomach acids and the digestive process, the microorganisms move through the stomach to the intestinal tract where they form colonies along the intestinal walls. HSOs™ multiply in the intestines and actually compete with harmful bacteria and yeasts for receptor sites, crowding out the pathogens and taking up residence. Once established, the organisms quickly begin producing the proper environment to absorb nutrients and help to re-establish the proper pH. According to early research and anecdotal evidence the following is a summary of the actions of HSOs™.

- HSOs™ work from the inside of the intestines dislodging accumulated decay on the walls and flushing out waste
- HSOs™ breaks down hydrocarbons. This process has a unique ability to split food into its most basic elements allowing almost total absorption through the digestive system. This increases overall nutrition and enhances cellular development
- HSOs™ produce specific proteins that act as antigens, encouraging the immune system to produce huge pools of un-coded antibodies. This increased production of antibodies may significantly boost the body's ability to ward off diseases
- HSOs™ are very aggressive against pathological molds, yeasts, fungi, bacteria, parasites and viruses
- HSOs™ work in symbiosis with somatic (tissue or organ) cells to metabolize proteins and eliminate toxic waste

- HSOs™ stimulate the body to produce natural alpha-interferon. Alpha-interferon is a potent immune system enhancer and inhibitor of viruses
- HSOs™ provide critical Lactoferrin supplementation. The microbes produce lactoferrin as a by-product of their metabolism. Lactoferrin is an iron binding protein essential for retrieving iron from foods

Probiotics Residential bacteria form colonies in the gastrointestinal tract, mouth, and vaginal tract. Transient bacteria are travelers that are just passing through. Friendly bacteria including *Lactobacillus acidophilus, Bifido-bacterium bifidum,* and *Lactobacillus bulgaricus* are the body's first line of defense against the potentially harmful microorganisms that are inhaled or ingested. Probiotics are another term for these friendly bacteria that live and work in the gastrointestinal tract. Think of them as a mighty bacterial army that defends the body against dangerous invaders. Having sufficient numbers of these friendly bacteria in residence can help prevent a wide range of health problems.

Bulgaricum* Bulgaricum (D-Lactobacillus bulgaricus, L.B. 51 strain (researched for the past 30 years), is a transient bacteria that has a catalytic-like action on Lactobacillus acidophilus and Bifidobacterium bifidum and is an efficient immune stimulant. It enhances the body's ability to metabolize lactose and other milk products, digest carbohydrates and proteins and also supports the body's ability to deal with heartburn, acid indigestion, food poisoning and acid reflux.

Not all probiotics are the same. Check the label for the presence of FOS: Fructooligosaccharides are a class of simple carbohydrates found naturally in plants like the Jerusalem artichoke. Extracting FOS from the heart of the Jerusalem artichoke yields natural FOS at up to 70 per cent. However, a Japanese chemical process uses the action of a fungal enzyme to turn white, bleached cane sugar into an artificial FOS resulting in a 98% yield. Since a 98% yield is commercially more attractive, virtually all FOS added to probiotic products in the U.S. are produced by this artificial process. For this reason we strongly recommend Natren brand which does not use this sweetener.

Three-in-One Dairy and Dairy-Free Natren®'s Healthy Trinity® capsules take probiotics to the next level of effectiveness with a simplified system that is both easy to use and understand. Healthy Trinity® capsules contain all three of the most potent super strains of beneficial bacteria: Lactobacillus acidophilus, NAS adhesion super strain, 5 billion cfu per capsule; adult specific Bifidobacterium bifidum, Malyoth super strain, 20 billion cfu per capsule; and Lactobacillus bulgaricus LB-51 champion transient super strain, 5 billion cfu per capsule. These amazing super strains may also be found in Natren®'s other Healthy Trinity® powders or capsules: Megadophilus®, Bifido Factor® and Digesta-Lac®.

Special Delivery System Ensures Potency

- Natren®'s dairy-free oil matrix complex keeps Healthy Trinity®'s targeted microorganisms separated and non competitive
- This first-of-its-kind delivery system utilizes sunflower oil and Vitamin E, which have all of the oxygen and water removed to create a totally anaerobic environment, (ideal for keeping the bacteria in a state of arrested growth, until it is introduced into the system and can be used most efficiently)
- This system ensures the microorganisms survive exposure to the stomach's gastric juices, thus offering maximum benefits to the small and large intestines

Usage instructions: Healthy Trinity® oil matrix capsules are formulated to be taken with a meal to enhance digestion, but may be taken at any time. Healthy Trinity® should be taken with room temperature, filtered (non-chlorinated) water. Healthy Trinity® powders should be mixed together in approximately 6 to 8 oz. of room temperature, filtered (un-chlorinated) water. The powders are formulated to be taken approximately 20-30 minutes before meals to enhance digestion, but may be taken at any time. If you are experiencing stomach upset, the mixture may be sipped throughout the day. Both capsules and powders should be taken at least 2 hours after consuming herbs (i.e., garlic and Echinacea) and prescription drugs (antibiotics). Some herbs and all antibiotics will eliminate not only undesirable, but beneficial bacteria as well.

Nutritional Action:

- Helps deter yeast overgrowth (Candida)
- Aids in lactose metabolism and enhances digestion of milk products
- May improve nutrient absorption
- Helps normalize elimination problems
- May block the attachment of bad bacteria in the urinary tract, including the vagina
- Helps alleviate gas, bloating and upper G.I. problems
- Produces hydrogen peroxide H2O2 — found necessary to inhibit vaginal yeast
- Neutralizes the formation of toxins
- Assists in cholesterol management
- Protects the walls of the large intestine from colonization by invading bacteria or yeast
- Inhibits bacteria, which can alter nitrates into potentially harmful nitrites; Supports healthy liver function
- Helps to promote regularity
- Encourages an acidic intestinal environment, which inhibits less desirable microorganisms
- Contributes to the growth and viability of beneficial resident microorganisms (*Lactobacillus acidophilus, Bifidobacterium bifidum,* etc.) by supporting their growth and activity
- Helps the body digest complex carbohydrates and proteins

- Helps to increase the bioavailability of minerals, especially calcium. The absorption is doubly important in lactose-intolerant individuals who may also experience a deficiency of dietary calcium
- May also produce antimicrobial substances antagonistic to various bad bacteria
- Produces B vitamins

> *Additional information and product purchases are available from:*
> Natren
> 1-800-992-3323
> *www.natren.com*

CLEANSING THE SMALL AND LARGE INTESTINE

Spanish Black Radish* Spanish Black Radish, a member of the brassica family, protects against free radicals — highly unstable molecules that can affect cells and genetic material. Spanish Black Radish is an excellent source of sulfur and is also beneficial in the healthy functioning of the gastrointestinal tract. This product also stimulates the body's own system for neutralizing harmful substances. Components such as indole-3-carbinol and sulforaphene are found in Spanish black radish. These two substances stimulate two of the body's most powerful detoxification mechanisms – the cytochrome p450 and the Phase II enzyme systems – the body's biochemical pathways for converting toxins into harmless or easily excretable substances.

Vegetarian product — 90 tablets

Available from: ICNR, Inc. 1-800-272-2323 or order at: *www.icnr.com*

Okra Pepsin E3 Allantoin, a primary ingredient in Okra Pepsin E3, promotes skin health. The properties of the combined nutrients in Okra Pepsin E3 also give this product bowel-cleansing capabilities. It digests the mucus that coats the walls of the small intestine. Certain foods, such as pasteurized milk and many cooked foods, cause the mucus buildup on the wall of the small intestine whereas raw foods do not cause this mucus buildup. The mucus coats the villi on the wall of the small intestine preventing absorption of nutrients from the digested food, which is primarily liquid. The mucus blockage varies with different people. Sometimes it blocks minerals and larger molecules only, while in other people it partially blocks all nutrients. Almost no nutrition can get through to the body. The consequences of a mucous, coated intestine are poor or little absorption of vitamins and or food and the possibility of slow starvation. That would lead to more of the pancreatic enzymes being used to digest protein even though it could not be properly absorbed. When all the pancreatic enzymes are used up, there are none left in the blood to destroy cancer cells. The okra tends to stick the pepsin enzyme to the mucus on the intestinal wall long enough to digest some of the mucus. The E-3 is a powerful tissue repair factor.

The Okra Pepsin E3 is indicated for both underweight and overweight people. In both cases nutrients are not being absorbed. Even if they are taking enzymes to digest the food they eat, they absorb only the smaller carbohydrate molecules while the larger protein molecules are blocked. In underweight people the carbohydrates are used efficiently (burned for energy, not turned into fat), but the person becomes thin as they lose muscle mass from lack of protein absorption. In overweight people the carbohydrates are not used efficiently (they are turned into fat), and this causes the person to become overweight as they also lose muscle mass. Available from: ICNR, Inc. 1-800-272-2323 or order on line at: *www.icnr.com*. *Size:* either 40 or 150 capsules; *Ingredients:* Okra, Tillandsia usneoides extract, bovine orchic extract, pepsin (1:10,000), carbamide, alginic acid, and allantoin.

INTESTINAL OBSTRUCTION

Doctor William Donald Kelly in his book, *Do-it-Yourself Book* One Answer To Cancer (*www.drkelley.com/CANLIVER55.html*) accurately describes the issues regarding intestinal blockage.

"Occasionally, the intestinal tract will become obstructed. Usually under these circumstances, no food or feces will come through. After a few days, one becomes extremely nauseated and starts vomiting. He or she will be very sick and will normally run a high temperature. This should be watched quite carefully, for in such cases immediate emergency treatment is absolutely necessary.

"One should never allow themselves to become extremely toxic. But, in order to distinguish between a healing toxic reaction and an intestinal obstruction, as soon as nausea or vomiting develops and no food is passing through, all supplements and food should be stopped for 5 days. Water and juice may be taken during this time.

"If there is no vomiting, food is passing through, and the temperature remains below 100 degrees, the diet and normal routine may be resumed, as one may assume there is no obstruction.

"A point to remember is that one shouldn't fail to cycle off the supplements routinely before reaching such a state of toxicity!

"If, during the 5 days off the supplements with no solid food intake, one begins to vomit and has abdominal pain with high temperature, a physician should check for intestinal obstruction."

CLEANSING THE KIDNEYS

Arginex® Arginex® is a product formulated to support the cleansing ability of the kidneys. *Content:* 90 Tablets

Available from: ICNR, Inc. 1-800-272-2323 or order on line at: *www.icnr.com*.

The kidneys are vital organs of detoxification. They filter approximately 4,000 quarts of blood daily. The metabolic wastes, largely urea, are eliminated and the acid/alkaline balance maintained. Many drugs are eliminated through the kidneys, especially the common pain killing or NSAID drugs that can be extremely damaging to these organs. Such drugs include, Tylenol, Advil, Nuprin and aspirin. Medical literature states that taking 5000 doses of a NSAID drug will cause irreversible kidney damage. Unfortunately, patients do not experience any symptoms from kidney function loss until 90% of the function is gone, and then the damage is irreversible.

The kidneys should be flushed each day with liberal quantities of fluid, either Reverse Osmosis filtered water, distilled water or fresh fruit and vegetable juices (preferably organic). Parsley tea is excellent for strengthening the kidneys. Those with kidney problems should avoid ordinary commercial teas and coffee. Herbal teas are acceptable.

For those who tend to retain fluid, Boswellia Complex is an excellent herbal supplement that functions as a diuretic. Steeping fresh ginger for 30 minutes in boiled distilled water can make an excellent diuretic tea. In extreme fluid retention, a physician may have to prescribe a diuretic drug. The doctor will normally increase the intake of potassium and B1 (thiamin) to compensate for their drug induced loss.

In kidney disease the protein intake should be limited and a protomorphagen (genetic blueprint) product, Renatrophin PMG, should be used to help rebuild the kidney.

Renatrophin PMG® contains Protomorphagen™ extracts, which are uniquely derived nucleoprotein-mineral extracts that support cellular health. Bovine kidney PMG™ extract helps to support healthy kidney gland function. Content: 90 Tablets; Available from: ICNR, Inc. 1-800-272-2323 or order on line at: *www.icnr.com*.

CLEANSING THE GALLBLADDER

The bile acts as a carrier for all liver wastes. It is also essential for the proper digestion and assimilation of fats and all fat-soluble nutrients such as vitamins A, D, E, K, lecithin, and essential fatty acids. The gallbladder is a hollow muscular organ, which stores and concentrates bile. When food is ingested, especially if it contains fats or oils, the gallbladder is stimulated to contract and should freely expel its contents into the small intestine to emulsify fatty nutrients for proper absorption, and to allow poisonous wastes, which the liver has removed from the body, to be eliminated through the intestines.

Patients with cancer invariably have toxic livers and thick bile, which does not flow easily through the bile ducts. A key to a successful gallbladder flush is in the preparation. It is strongly recommended that preliminary steps be taken:

- Cleanse the kidneys
- Clean out the intestines
- Remove all mercury fillings and any infections in the jaw bone

- Do a parasite cleanse
- Soften any gallstones with apple juice (malic acid), Choline (fraction of the B-complex vitamins- three to five tablets before each meal) and AF Betafood® (made from red beets and beet tops- three to five tablets before each meal). This program should be used for six to eight weeks prior to carrying out the gallbladder flush.

There are several very good gallbladder flush programs available. The following web sites provide all the detailed information.

www.curezone.com/cleanse/liver/huldas_recipe.asp

www.curezone.com/cleanse/liver/kelley.asp

www.curezone.com/cleanse/liver/liver_flush_protocol_ortophospho.asp

No matter which protocol is used sickness may result from the process. The more toxic the individual the greater the number and intensity of symptoms. Unfortunately this is part of the healing process. The typical major reactions include nausea, diarrhea, vomiting, profuse sweating, dizziness, weakness and headache. Stopping consumption of all processed foods can reduce these symptoms and eating mainly steamed organic fresh vegetables and steroid and antibiotic-free chicken and beef. Eating wholesome food will start the cleansing process. Cleaning out the intestines with high fiber and Herbal C formula will take the burden off the liver/gallbladder and speed the liver's ability to dump the poisons. Taking the appropriate supplements (antioxidants, vitamins, enzymes, herbs, homeopathics, etc.) will help neutralize many of the poisons.

CLEANSING THE LUNGS

The blood cleanses itself of carbonic acid via the exchange of gases in the lungs. The most significant exchange is the removal of carbonic acid and the flow of oxygen into the blood. The lungs give off many other gaseous wastes. Frequently after the start of the detoxification the patient may notice a foul body and breath odor. No attempt to mask this problem (breath mints, toothpaste or mouthwash) will remove it. This process will continue until the noxious substances have left the body.

Mucus-forming foods such as dairy products, with the exception of butter and cream, and baked flour products should be avoided. Anti-mucus foods such as raw onions and garlic, cayenne pepper, freshly ground black pepper, fresh ginger, and horseradish or diakon (Japanese radish) should be eaten liberally.

CLEANSING THE SKIN

Many toxic substances are eliminated through the skin, which is the second biggest excretory gland of the body. Lightly brushing the skin with a loofah sponge stimulates blood and lymphatic circulation and removes dead cells to promote elimination. Brush feet and upwards towards the heart, since it is important to follow the flow of lymphatic fluid. Brush from the fingertips up to the shoulders and toward the heart. Use small strokes and gentle pressure. Avoid the facial area and irritated skin. Skin brushing can easily be incorporated into a daily routine when performed before showering or bathing.

Alternating between hot and cold-water helps increase circulation, promotes detoxification and strengthens the immune system. This helps bring nutrients, oxygen and immune cells to damaged and stressed tissues and carries away metabolic waste, inflammatory by-products and other toxic substances. Start with three minutes of hot water followed by less than one minute of cold water. Repeat this pattern at least once, always finishing with cold (e.g. 3 minutes hot — 1 minute cold — 3 minutes hot — 1 minute cold). This process stimulates the autonomic nervous system: hot (parasympathetic) and cold (sympathetic).

Another approach to drawing out toxins through the skin is to take an Epsom salt bath. These baths are especially beneficial during a "healing crisis" when feeling especially toxic and ill. Such a bath works best after the skin brushing. Add 4 or more cups of Epsom salt to a tub filled with warm to hot water. Make sure contents are completely dissolved. The magnesium in the Epsom salts is effective in relaxing tense, sore muscles.

"Natural, healthy food begets health. Divitalized, processed and chemicalized food begets disease. No simpler truth exists. No greater lie is told than that to obscure the truth."

Lester Kessel (1926-1989)

Section 5

NUTRIENTS TO REGENERATE
YOUR BODY

In a perfect world all our food would have high energy levels, be pesticide and toxin free, and have maximum nutritional content. In the real world, our food starts decaying the moment it is harvested and each day of transit its energy level decreases and the contents continue to decay. In addition, the soils in which the crops are grown are depleted of vital nutrients so that the plants are deficient. This deplorable state of our soil erosion started after World War II when fertilizer companies pushed the concept that synthetic fertilizers would improve food production and save costs. The end result has been deficient soils and food, and a scourge of degenerative diseases that medicine believes it can correct through genetic engineering.

Since it is extremely difficult for most people to access organically grown food and natural food restaurants, it is an absolute necessity to supplement the diet with broad based food concentrates and eliminate or greatly reduce the intake of toxic foods. The more ill the patient the greater the need for full and strict compliance to resolve their health issues.

The following recommendations are based on clinical experience. These choices are by no means all that are available but have been chosen for their extreme high quality and wide range of essential food based nutrients. As with all nutrients, these recommendations must be tested for biocompatibility. *One of the major discoveries that this author has gleaned from successfully reversing ovarian cancer was that selecting biocompatible nutrients speeds up the healing process.* The underlying common denominator is the nutrients ability to restore the energy balance of the patient's body. In the quest to find the "magic bullets" of health many protocols are offered by well meaning people and health care practitioners alike. Consider all these recommendations and if they prove compatible add to the daily regimen.

PERFECT FOOD*

Perfect Food™ contains the highest quality ingredients. Many other products use large amounts of inexpensive ingredients such as lecithin, apple fiber and flax seed meal. While these compounds do provide some benefit, they are not nearly as beneficial as nutrient rich whole foods such as greens. These filler ingredients significantly reduce the manufacturer's cost of the product. Considering the cost of green super foods, inexpensive ingredients used as fillers such as lecithin, apple fiber, rice bran and flax meal should not represent more than 10% of the product. If you look at the competing brands, the aforementioned ingredients typically make up over 30% of the product by weight. Perfect Food™ contains over 8500mg of highly concentrated absorbable green foods with no filler ingredients. Perfect Food™ is high in nutrition and low in calories, making it ideal for those on low carbohydrate diets. Perfect Food™ is designed to provide the highest quality vegetable nutrition to everyone.

Ingredients *Green Super Foods:* Kamut Grass, Wheat Grass, Barley Grass, Oat Grass, Alfalfa Grass, Spirulina, Chlorella, Dunaliella, Kelp and Dulse. Green Super Foods are a rich source of vitamins, minerals, enzymes, amino acids, chlorophyll and antioxidants. (Gluten and Phytate free)

Vegetables Carrot Juice, Beet Juice, Tomato Juice, Sweet Potato, Brocolli, Kale, Cabbage, Cauliflower, Brussels Sprouts, Parsley, Spinach, Asparagus, Celery, Cucumber, Green Pepper, Garlic, Ginger and Onion. Vegetables are nature's richest sources of phytochemicals including lycopene, sulforophane, allicin and bioflavonoids.

Grains and Seeds Flax Seeds, Sesame Seeds, Sunflower Seeds, Pumpkin Seeds, Chia Seeds Garbanzo Beans, Red Lentils, Soy Beans, Kidney Beans, Azuki Beans, Oats, Barley, Rye, Millet, Brown Rice, Maize and Buckwheat (Gluten and Phytate Free). Easily digestible grains, seeds and legumes provide vitamins such as B complex and vitamin E, Isoflavones, fiber and essential fatty acids including Omega 3 and 6.

Acerola Cherry Nature's richest source of vitamin C. Vitamin C is crucial as a premier antioxidant and is important for the health of the immune system.

CERTIFIED ORGANIC

Poten-Zyme™ Process The nutrient rich superfoods contained in Perfect Food™ are pre-digested using the proprietary Poten-Zyme™ process. The Poten-Zyme™ process is an ancient bio fermentation process using beneficial microorgainisms (probiotics) and their enzymes to gently break down foods into their basic elements. Poten-Zyme™ neutralizes nutrient inhibitors found in foods such as grains, seeds and legumes. Many people with sensitive digestive systems have a tough time obtaining nutrition from these sometimes difficult to digest foods. Poten-Zyme™ solves that problem. Poten-Zyme™ creates and liberates valuable compounds within the foods including: enzymes, antioxidants, beta glucans, and phytosterols. Poten-Zyme™ enhances the nutritional value of food while making it much easier to digest. This assures the Perfect Food™ user more complete absorption and delivery of nutrients at the cellular level. Some of the longest living and healthiest people in history have relied on fermented foods such as yogurt, kefir, miso and sauerkraut to supply them with much needed nutrition and aid in digestion. Unlike other products, the probiotics and enzymes contained in Perfect Food™ are created within the foods themselves. Perfect Food™ provides probiotics, enzymes and phytonutrients in one whole food package. Where other super foods isolate, Perfect Food™ completes. For product information check Garden of Life web site: *www.gardenoflifeusa.com*

Pure Synergy™* The Synergy Company™, deeply respects and trusts the innate wisdom of nature. They know that the health-enhancing nourishment and life energy contained in whole foods cannot ever be fully replicated by a synthesized chemical created in a test tube. So why do companies use synthetic chemicals? They cost considerably less — using synthetic chemicals is an easy way to cut corners. By nature, whole-food ingredients are variable, so it can be challenging and costly to ensure their consistent potency and quality. Most companies are not willing to invest in developing and maintaining the necessary technologies and standards that ensure safe and consistently potent products. However, because the benefits from consuming whole-food supplements are so superior, they have perfected many 100% natural growing, concentrating, processing and packaging technologies to overcome these challenges.

The Synergy Company™, specializes in safely capturing, concentrating and preserving all the vitality found in nutrient-rich foods to create unique, unsurpassed formulas bursting with all the goodness nature intended. And they do it naturally! There are no synthetic or isolated chemicals in any of their products, just pure, wholesome ingredients to restore and regenerate vitality and a sense of well-being. Optimally nourished, bodies naturally revitalize and radiate a glowing wellness.

PHYTONUTRIENTS PROVIDE VITAL HEALTH-PROTECTIVE BENEFITS?

"Scientists and researchers are now recommending nine servings a day of fruits and vegetables. Why so much? Greens and fruits are abundant sources of vitamins and minerals, but, more importantly, they are phytonutrient powerhouses. The phytonutrient compounds that function as a plant's immune system offer substantial antioxidant and detoxifying benefits. Chlorophyll, carotenes, lutein, bioflavonoids, anthocyanins, proanthocyanins and phycocyanins are responsible for many of the health-protective benefits in diets rich in fruits and vegetables.

Pure Synergy™ contains over seventy vital phytonutrients. Grass juices, algae, sea vegetables, spinach, collards, kale and berries are the richest known sources of many of these precious compounds. More important, *Pure Synergy*™ provides these phytonutrients in their natural, synergistic food form. This means that the phytonutrients, vitamins and minerals contained in *Pure Synergy*™ enhance and support each other's activity, providing protective, regenerative and strengthening benefits to you! *Pure Synergy*™*'s* cleansing and regenerative grass juices, algae, seaweeds and enzymes are combined with protective fruits and berries and restorative, adaptogenic herbs and mushrooms to enhance natural detoxification and the radiant energy that results from genuine well-being. Unlike many other products there are no fillers or bulking agents (whole grasses, apple fiber or pectin, rice bran, flax or maltodextrin), which dilute nutritional potency and are a potential source of genetically modified material. Because the cellulose fiber in whole grass is indigestible, it prevents the grass's valuable phytonutrients from being released in the digestive system. For this reason, Pure Synergy™ uses *only grass juices.* In every spoonful of *Pure Synergy*™*,* there are densely packed nutrients that intensely nourish and strengthen every system in the body, resulting in sustained energy, enhanced recovery, mental clarity and overall well-being!

Pure Synergy™ is special not only because of its extraordinary formula, but also because it is meticulously cultivated to protect all its precious constituents. The company works closely with certified organic growers to ensure the optimal development of enzymes and beneficial phytonutrients in *Pure Synergy's* ingredients. These extraordinary herbs and other foods are harvested at their peak of potency and immediately concentrated and dried by utilizing proprietary cool-temperature processes that preserve their energetic and nutritional integrity. Studies have shown that these unique technologies offer unprecedented protection of the enzymes and other valuable phytonutrient constituents. The Ultra Fresh Packaging™ further protects *Pure Synergy*™ from damaging light, oxygen and moisture after bottling." Michael May founder and CEO.

All *Pure Synergy's* ingredients are comprehensively tested, and this superior product is made at *The Synergy Company's* own award-winning facility, that is certified to manufacture organic and kosher products.

Eating is such an ordinary part of our daily lives that we often lose sight of its enormous importance. Our need for healthy food goes far beyond our requirement for the fuel provided by calories. The vital health-enhancing vitamins, minerals, enzymes, phytonutrients and other compounds found in whole, unprocessed foods, such as *Pure Synergy*™, provide the components our cells require to carry out their life-sustaining work. This work includes fighting off infection; pumping blood; digesting and absorbing nutrients; carrying neural signals in the brain; facilitating procreation; rebuilding bone, connective tissue and skin; and contracting and relaxing muscles. If we don't receive adequate amounts of these essential compounds, literally every cell in our body is adversely affected because, like a line of dominos falling, adverse effects travel from one system in the body to another. This process is often subtle at first and slow to manifest. In fact, research shows that there is usually a 10- to 20-year period of gradual deterioration in our bodies before a diagnosable health challenge develops. While this information may sound frightening, *it is actually tremendously empowering*. During that 10-to 20-year period, our lifestyle and dietary choices are extremely important because they can inhibit this deterioration. *The choices you make today do impact your life tomorrow!*

Mitchell M. May, Ph.D.
Founder and CEO
The Synergy Company™

HOW TO USE PURE SYNERGY PROPERLY

Pure Synergy™ can be mixed with a variety of liquids. Many people choose pure, filtered water; others use juice or a combination of juice and water. Pour 8 to 10 ounces of liquid into a jar or glass with a tight-fitting lid, and add *Pure Synergy*™. Put the lid on the jar or glass, and shake well. *Pure Synergy*™ is ready to drink! Lump alert: Please do not try to stir your *Pure Synergy*™ into liquid — it will be lumpy! Shaking or blending ensures a smooth beverage.

Open Pure Synergy™ *gently*. To protect the precious phytonutrients in *Pure Synergy*™ from heat, light and oxygen, the company seals the bottle using the state-of-the-art *Ultra Fresh Packaging*™ system. This unique system creates a pressurized and highly protective oxygen-free environment inside the sealed bottle. When *Pure Synergy*™ is opened there is a whooshing, suction noise as the air pressure equalizes between the bottle and the surrounding environment. In some cases, depending on altitude and other atmospheric conditions, the pressure differential between the bottle and the surrounding environment is greater and results in a loud popping noise when the seal is peeled off! This is a sign the product is absolutely fresh. Prick the seal on a bottle of *Pure Synergy*™ bottle with a pin or knife tip and then remove the seal.

Begin gradually. The daily serving of *Pure Synergy*™ is one heaping tablespoon. However, when adding *Pure Synergy*™ to the diet for the first time, please begin slowly. This allows the body to comfortably acclimate to a deeper level of nutrition. We suggest beginning with one-quarter to one teaspoon of *Pure Synergy*™ and gradually increasing to one heaping tablespoon or more daily.

Drink Pure Synergy™ *on an empty stomach.* The vital nutrients and phytonutrients in *Pure Synergy*™ are most easily absorbed if consumed on an empty stomach. Many people find it convenient to drink *Pure Synergy* first thing in the morning and then wait at least 30 minutes before consuming any other food.

Drink plenty of water. Water is essential to optimal health. Drink 8 to 10 glasses of pure, filtered water throughout the day. Coffee, juice and soda pop do not count as water! *Protect Pure Synergy*™. An unopened bottle of *Pure Synergy*™ can be kept in any dark, cool location, such as a cupboard, drawer or closet, for up to five years. Please keep opened bottles of *Pure Synergy*™ in the freezer or refrigerator. It will last about three months in the refrigerator, and six months in the freezer. Available from: ICNR, Inc. 1-800-272-2323 or order on line at: *www.icnr.com.*

SP Complete™ SP Complete™ is a whole food and botanical supplement that mixes with water to make a nutritious supplement shake — completely portable for today's busy schedules. It offers a balance of essential macro- and micronutrients from plant sources in a highly bio-available form. The natural whole food and botanical ingredients used to formulate SP Complete™ support healthy cardiovascular, digestive, and nervous system function, and deliver powerful antioxidant protection to promote cellular health. Whether taken alone or before meals, a supplement shake made with SP Complete™ provides essential vitamins and minerals to the body during purification. In addition, SP Complete™ can be used outside of the purification program to replace vital nutrients often lost during the refining process.

Proprietary Blend: 25 g Whey protein powder, flax meal powder, brown rice protein powder, calcium citrate, magnesium citrate, buckwheat juice powder, Brussels sprouts powder, kale powder, choline bitartrate, inositol, barley grass juice powder, alfalfa sprout powder, Ginkgo biloba extract (24% flavone glycosides, 6% terpene lactones), soy bean lecithin powder, milk thistle extract (80% Silymarins), gotu kola powder, Ginkgo biloba leaf powder, grape seed extract (includes Masquelier's® OPC-85; 98% total phenolic compounds; 65% proanthocyanidins), carrot powder, green tea leaf powder, red wine extract (95% total phenols) green tea extract (50% poly phenols), and standardized bilberry extract (25% anthocyanosides). Available from: ICNR, Inc. 1-800-272-2323 or order on line at: *www.icnr.com.*

DIETARY REGIMES

There are numerous dietary concepts, which one can incorporate into their healing program. It is not the goal of this book to provide an in depth discussion of each one but to provide a guide for the patient and their health care practitioner to make choices.

The concept of Metabolic Typing discussed in section 6 was used because in my clinical experience it was a logical and practical approach to implement. The ultimate goal was to rebalance the autonomic nervous system for optimal body function. Once the basics are understood it is relatively easy to follow, and the food choices are readily available with no major changes in cooking style required.

The following list provides major and miscellaneous schools of thought in specific dietary programs:

- Macrobiotics
- Ayurvedic
- Vegetarianism
- Vegan
- Pritikin Diet
- Atkins Diet
- Dr. Berger's Power Immune Diet
- Zone Diet
- Eat Right For Your Type
- Chinese System of Food Cures
- Life Extension
- Dr. Abravanel's Body Type Diet

The goal of any dietary approach should be to provide wholesome foods, preferably organic, that help repair the body, boost the immune system, reduce toxicity, supply nutrients that are physiologically needed (like animal protein for specific metabolic types), balance the autonomic nervous system and provide modifications to meet individual needs. If these criteria are met the patient has a much better chance of reversing their cancer.

Foods and products that must be stopped immediately Traditional medicine knows nothing about the impact foods have on creating the environment for cancer to grow. This is routinely witnessed on the 11 o'clock news when a lifeless child who is being destroyed by chemotherapy is given a milkshake to soothe their misery. In the view of Josef Issels, MD, a German cancer researcher, "Cancer is primarily a generalized disease, providing the substrate which allows the tumor to develop as the most important symptom or sign. This means that a tumor can only develop in a diseased organism." What Dr. Issels realized as far back as the 1950's is that in order to regenerate the body, one must stop eating chemicalized, devitalized "foods" and increase consumption of unadulterated foods to promote an environment in which cancer cannot grow.

These foods provide a major influence on cancer and should not be eaten:

Sugar Other than supplying pure calories, white sugar is totally devoid of nutritional value and *must not be ingested by cancer patients!*

- Processed sugar *blocks* the absorption of calcium. Four ounces of sugar will depress the calcium level for six days. Calcium is crucial in maintaining an alkaline environment within cells. The alkalinity increases oxygen and prevents the genetic code from being altered. Both processes help reduce the chances for cancer.

- Processed sugar produces a low oxygen environment. Cancer thrives on low oxygen and is one of the conditions that must be present for its growth.

- Processed sugar is extremely acidic. An acidic environment also contributes to low oxygen and to production of lactic acid instead of four essential amino acids that repair the genetic code.

- Too much processed sugar is the death of the immune system. It interrupts the Kreb's energy cycle, which in turn suppresses the immune system's ability to manufacture killer cells and antibodies.

- Processed sugar depletes B vitamins, which are needed to detoxify the liver. The liver is the most important organ when it comes to healing the body.

- Processed sugar stimulates production of insulin. Cancer cells have ten times more insulin receptors than normal cells enabling influx of calories to meet their rapid growth.

Aspartame This artificial sweetener is one of the more toxic substances on the market. At 86°F aspartame breaks down into formic acid, wood alcohol and formaldehyde. These same three components plus a compound called DKP, which may cause brain tumors, occur when aspartame is ingested. Wood alcohol and formaldehyde are potential carcinogenic substances.

Avoid all other sugar substitutes with the exception of Stevia, a natural sweetener derived from the bark and leaves of a South American tree. Stevia has been used as a commercial sweetener in soft drinks in Japan since the 1960's with no reported ill effects.

Salt Table salt is 99% pure sodium chloride compared to sea salt, which are 78% sodium chloride plus trace minerals. Salt consumption causes dehydration, concentrating toxins within tissues, which ultimately causes cells to die.

Caffeine This seemingly innocuous drug acts as a diuretic to flush minerals out of the body. Caffeine also causes a narrowing of the blood vessels decreasing blood supply to essential organs and other sites in the body. This addictive drug also over stimulates the sympathetic nervous system.

Milk Humans are the only species that drink milk after they are weaned. There are many problems with milk. Cow's milk is too acidic and reduces the oxygen content of fluids, tissues and organs. Also, cow's milk contains growth hormones as well as female sex hormones, which may stimulate the growth of tumors. Like meat, cows' milk has too high a protein content, requiring too many pancreatic enzymes for digestion. Furthermore pasteurization compounds the problem as it denatures the protein making its contents more of a waste product. A greater concern is the presence of antibiotics and steroids in milk that suppress the body's immune system as well as create superbugs as the pathogens develop resistance to the drugs.

Coffee The coffee bean, like the peanut, cleanses the soil of toxic chemicals. According to Kay Munsen, a nutritionist at Iowa State University, there are 393 chemical compounds in coffee. *Listed below are some of the more harmful substances:*

- Acetone
- Caffeine
- Methylfuran
- Butanol
- Methyl acetate
- Methanol
- Isoprene
- Furan
- Acetaldehyde
- Methylglyoxal
- Ethanol
- Diacetyl
- Methyl Formate
- Methylbutanol
- Dimethyl sulfide
- Dicarbonyl-aldehyde

Peanuts The presence of aflatoxins, known carcinogens, makes this food potentially toxic.

Non-Organic Red Meats and Poultry Commercially raised beef and poultry are contaminated with antibiotics, steroids and pesticides.

Processed lunch meats These foods are loaded with preservatives, coloring agents and in some cases scraps (bones and body parts) as fillers.

- Avoid *all* irradiated and genetically altered foods!
- Avoid cooking any food even heating water with microwave units.
- Avoid sautéing foods in oils. Heating the best oil will transform it into a trans-fatty acid. It is best to sauté in water and then add the oil.

Bacon This traditional American breakfast food contains dimethyl nitrosamine, a cancer causing substance.

Barbequing Smoking accelerates lipid peroxidation of unsaturated fats in fish and the oxidation of cholesterol in meats. The smoking process creates polycyclic aromatic hydrocarbons, a hazardous substance.

White bread There is very little nutritional value in bleached flower products that have the nutrients milled out. The synthetic vitamins replaced to fortify the paste will not meet the body's real needs.

White Rice This processed food is a pure starch and devoid of essential nutrients.

Sodas and other carbonated drinks Besides being loaded with corn syrup, manufacturers make the water in the drink very acidic (pH2.6) to increase carbonation and shelf life. Virtually nothing can grow in an acidic solution.

Processed lunch meats These foods are loaded with preservatives, coloring agents and in some cases scraps (bones and body parts) as fillers.

Dried Breakfast Cereals The milling process removes most of the essential vitamins, minerals, oils and fiber.

Shellfish This seafood has a greater propensity of being contaminated with bacteria.

Non-Organically Grown Fruits and Vegetables Commercially grown fruits and vegetables, especially produce from South America, are contaminated with pesticides, herbicides, fungicides, arsenic and other poisonous substances. You can obtain a comprehensive list of pesticides found in food at the following web site: *www.foodnews.org/*

Sources for organic foods The LocalHarvest map makes it easy to find family farms, farmers markets and other sources of sustainably grown food in your area. *www.localharvest.org/*

Alcohol (beer, wine and hard liquor) Preliminary studies show that alcohol may affect cancer development at the genetic level by affecting oncogenes at the initiation and developmental stages of cancer. It has been suggested that acetaldehyde, a product of alcohol metabolism, impairs a cell's natural ability to repair its DNA, resulting in a greater likelihood that mutations causing cancer initiation will occur (*Espina, N.*; Lima, V.; Lieber, C.S.; and Garro, A.J. In vitro and in vivo inhibitory effect of ethanol and acetaldehyde on methylguanine transferase. *Carcinogenesis* 9(5):761-766, 1988 (*Kharbanda, S.*; Nakamura, T.; and Kufe, D. Induction of the c-jun proto-oncogene by a protein kinase C-dependent mechanism during exposure of human epidermal keratinocytes to ethanol. *Biochemical Pharmacology* 45(3):675-681, 1993). It has recently been suggested that alcohol exposure may result in over expression of certain oncogenes in human cells triggering cancer promotion).

Alcohol as a co-carcinogen. Although there is no evidence that alcohol itself is a carcinogen, alcohol may act as a co-carcinogen by enhancing the carcinogenic effects of other chemicals. Studies indicate that alcohol enhances tobacco's ability to stimulate tumor formation in rats (29). In humans, the risk for mouth, tracheal, and esophageal cancer is 35 times greater for people who both smoke and drink than for people who neither smoke nor drink (30), implying a cocarcinogenic interaction between alcohol and tobacco-related carcinogens (*Garro, A.J.*, and Lieber, C.S. Alcohol and cancer. *Annual Review of Pharmacology and Toxicology* 30:219-249, 1990.).

Alcohol's co-carcinogenic effect may be explained by its interaction with certain enzymes. Some enzymes that normally help to detoxify substances that enter the body can also increase the toxicity of some carcinogens. One of these enzymes is called cytochrome P-450 (*Seitz, H.K.*, and Osswald, B. Effect of ethanol on procarcinogen activation. In: Watson, R.R., ed. *Alcohol and Cancer.* Boca Raton, FL: CRC Press, 1992. pp. 55-72.) and (*Garro, A.J.*; Espina, N.; and Lieber, C.S. Alcohol and cancer. *Alcohol Health & Research World* 16(1):81-86, 1992.. Dietary alcohol is able to induce cytochrome P-450 in the liver, lungs, esophagus, and intestines (*Farinati, F.*; Lieber, C.S.; and Garro, A.J. Effects of chronic ethanol consumption on carcinogen activating and detoxifying systems in rat upper alimentary tract tissue where alcohol-associated cancers occur. Alcoholism: *Clinical and Experimental Research* 13(3):357-360,1989.) Eventually, carcinogens such as those from tobacco and diet can become more potent as they, too, pass through the esophagus, lungs, intestines, and liver and encounter the activated enzyme. (*Farinati, F.*; Lieber, C.S.; and Garro, A.J. Effects of chronic ethanol consumption on carcinogen activating and detoxifying systems in rat upper alimentary tract tissue. Alcoholism: *Clinical and Experimental Research* 13(3):357-360, 1989.).

Nutrition: Chronic alcohol abuse may result in abnormalities in the way the body processes nutrients and may subsequently promote certain types of cancer. Reduced levels of iron, zinc, vitamin E, and some of the B vitamins, common in heavy drinkers, have been experimentally associated with some cancers (29). Also, levels of vitamin A, hypothesized to have anticancer properties (34), are severely depressed in the liver and esophagus of rats during chronic alcohol consumption (Mobarhan, S.; Layden, T.J.; Friedman, H.; Kunigk, A.; and Donahue, P. Depletion of liver and esophageal epithelium vitamin A after chronic moderate ethanol consumption in rats: Inverse relation to zinc nutriture.

Hepatology 6(4):615-621, 1986. *(36) Sato, M.*, and Lieber, C.S. Hepatic vitamin A depletion after chronic ethanol consumption in baboons and rats. *Journal of Nutrition* 111(11):2015-2023, 1991. *(37) Ziegler, R.G.* A review of epidemiologic evidence that carotenoids reduce the risk of cancer. *Journal of Nutrition* 119(1):116-122, 1989.).

A recent study indicates that as few as two drinks per day negates any beneficial effects of a "correct" diet on decreasing risk of colon cancer (38). Although the study suggests that a diet high in folic acid, a B vitamin found in fresh fruits and vegetables, decreases the risk for colon cancer, it also warns that alcohol consumption may counter this protective action and increase the risk for colon cancer by reducing folic acid levels.

Suppression of immune response. Alcoholism has been associated with suppression of the human immune system. Immune suppression makes chronic alcohol abusers more susceptible to various infectious diseases and, theoretically, to cancer (*Roselle, G.* Alcohol and the immune system. *Alcohol Health & Research World* 16(1):16-22, 1992).

Pork The internationally known researcher, Dr. Gaston Nassens, discovered that eating pork causes the cells of the blood to take on the characteristics of cancer for an eight-hour period. For an introduction to Dr. Gaston Nassens' work go to the following web site: *www.euroamericanhealth.com/gaston.html*

Snack Foods Many snack foods (potato chips, cookies, donuts, candies, cakes, etc.) are high in quantities of sugars, artificial colorings, preservatives and hydrogenated fats. The process of hydrogenation, the addition of hydrogen atoms to fatty-acid chains of polyunsaturates, is designed to increase the fat's stability and degree of hardness. Combing the hydrogen with polyunsaturates creates trans-fatty acids (TFA's), which can be extremely toxic. These trans-fatty acids are less digestible and metabolically more dangerous. TFA's linkages prevent the formation of bile in the liver from cholesterol with the end result of increased cholesterol levels.

Margarine and solid vegetable shortenings and synthetic fats (Olestra) These are solid trans-fatty acids, are difficult for the body to use in its regulatory machinery. The influx of these trans-fatty acids into the lymph and circulatory systems thickens these fluids increasing the stickiness factor of blood platelets. These TFA's do not supply electrons to the body cells. As a result of this loss of bipolarity, the course of growth is disturbed and cancers develop manifesting as tumors. The use of synthetic fats, like Olestra, prevents the absorption of fat-soluble vitamins and other valuable nutrients from the intestinal wall. They also are responsible for causing anal leakage.

Fast Foods These toxic, devitalized foods include: hamburger, hot dogs, wings, pizza, steak sandwiches, French fries, cheese wiz, cream cheese, onion rings, fried foods, milk shakes, hot chocolate, sugary desserts.

Bisphenol-A (BPA) Bisphenol-A was originally developed in the 1930's as a synthetic form of the female hormone estrogen. Later bisphenol-A was incorporated into plastic known as polycarbonate. However, not all of the BPA in polycarbonate fully "polymerizes" to form polycarbonate. Some remains "unreacted." As a result, concentrations of BPA in household products can be as much as 58 parts per million (according to FDA), a very high amount considering BPA's possible biological effects. Some of the unreacted BPA gets washed away in initial use and washings, but it can also migrate into the contents of the containers. If the containers are scratched, even more leaching can occur according to scientists at the University of Nagasaki, Japan. Bisphenol-A in baby bottles has been found to leach into the liquid when hot. The liquid in some cans of tinned vegetables have been found to contain both bisphenol-A, and the related chemical dimethyl bisphenol-A. The highest levels of bisphenol-A were found in cans of peas, with an average of 23 ug per can. Bisphenol-A was also found in the liquids of cans of artichokes, beans, mixed vegetables, corn and mushrooms. Eating foods like fried chicken, mountain cheese, and some species of fish will provide phenol exposure.

Fluoridated toothpaste/Fluoridated water The fluoride levels in toothpaste can range from 600 parts per million to as high as 1500 parts per million. Fluoride is a known carcinogen. *"In point of fact, fluoride causes more human cancer, and causes it faster, than any other chemical."* Dean Burk, Chief Chemist Emeritus, U.S. National Cancer Institute.
Burk's final statement on fluoridated water and its causal relationship between fluoridation and cancer death rate was, "It is concluded that artificial fluoridation appears to cause or induce about 20-30 excess deaths for every 100,000 persons exposed per year after about 15-20 years." To learn more about the dangers of fluoride go to the following web site: *www.nofish.org/new_page_3.htm*

Cosmetics, perfumed soaps and shampoos In general, beauty aids are loaded with chemical compounds that are potentially hazardous.

Underarm Deodorants Most commercial antiperspirants use aluminum to stop the perspiration. There are deodorants available that have no aluminum or other toxic chemicals. For more information on aluminum free deodorant and other products contact the Allergy Relief Shop, Inc. 1-800-626-2810. They also have a consultation line 1-423-494-4100.

The key points to remember are:

- Every thing in moderation
- Minimize any binging on processed foods
- Avoid over loading the system with toxic substances

"We are indeed much more than we eat, but what we eat can nevertheless help us to be much more than what we are."

Adelle Davis (1926-1989)

Section 6

METABOLIC TYPING AND DIETARY SCHEDULES

"Degenerative conditions account for well over 80% of all of the adverse conditions that afflict the peoples of our country. This means that only a little over 1 out of every 10 people that go to doctors has crises or infectious conditions that require — and respond to — allopathic applications. More and more people every year fall prey to degenerative conditions and, sadly, at younger and younger ages".

Statistics on degenerative diseases:

- Estimated 10 million hyperactive children with serious behavior problems.
- Estimated 16 million diabetics who require daily insulin injections.
- Estimated 25 million headache sufferers.
- Estimated 3 million adolescents clinically depressed.
- Estimated 2 million Americans suffering ulcerative colitis and irritable bowel syndrome.
- Over 50 million Americans suffering from sleep disorders
- More than 1 million people die annually from heart attacks.
- 55% of those who die from heart attack have hardening of the arteries.
- Estimated 300,000 die of stroke each year.
- Estimated by American Cancer Institute that by the year 2002 one in every two Americans will have cancer in their lifetime. In the 1930's the ratio was 3 out of one hundred got cancer.
- The US leads the world in the number of colon cancers and diverticulitis cases

ARTICLE BY HAROLD KRISTAL, DDS "Diseases once viewed, as accompaniments to old age are now commonplace in our children. Yet, currently, there is no orthodox cure for any degenerative disease. So-called alternative practitioners, as a group, fare little better. Even those who meet with "success" often find that when the therapy is stopped the condition returns and no real, lasting healing has taken place. Or they are baffled by the universal phenomena of failing to help the next patient with the same condition with the very protocol that worked so well for the former patient.

"We find ourselves trying futilely to absorb the avalanche of research in nutrition that has descended and promises to increase in volume. What are we to do with this blessing/curse? — The seemingly endless and often contradictory minutia of biochemical research? The problem is that there hasn't been a reference point, a framework in which to organize and understand the thousands upon thousands of research findings, many of, which are contradictory in nature. It's like an enormous jigsaw puzzle that arrives without the picture on the box. How do the pieces fit together? How can we possibly make sense, and make use, of this research?

"A PDR (Physician's Desk Reference) of nutrition? Just think about it for a moment. Even if it was possible to know the effects of every single vitamin, mineral, fatty acid, herb, etc., and then to organize them item by item, of what practical use would that be? How would we be any further along? We would still have 100's even 1000's of choices to make for each nutrient. And every day more and more effects are being found for every nutrient known to us, and this will continue ad infinitum. Even so, it is every practitioner's experience that what works for one patient does not work for another with the same condition.

"It should be obvious that the whole thing is one gigantic pool of randomized information that is only growing in complexity. And yet, this is precisely the path that researchers and practitioners are following. The wrong path was chosen and it is leading us deeper and deeper into the dark forest of confusion. The more research uncovers, the less clear the picture becomes. The wrong questions have been and are still being asked. Instead of seeking answers to the effects of biochemical substances on diseases, we need to turn our attention to understanding how nutrients affect individual metabolisms. Instead of thinking in terms of treating disease, we must learn to think in terms of building health and optimizing genetic functional capacity."

BIRTH OF METABOLIC TYPING

William Donald Kelly, DDS was a biologist, chemist, biochemist and pioneer in nutritional science. He is regarded as the "father of metabolic typing." In the mid-1960's he developed pancreatic cancer, which had metastasized to his liver, pelvis and other areas. Doctor Kelly was given only a few months to live. Out of necessity he put together an eclectic approach, which included diet, vitamins, minerals, enzymes and detoxification techniques. Doctor Kelly totally reversed his pancreatic cancer and is alive today some 42 years after he was given a death sentence by conventional medicine.

Kelly discovered the hard way that one approach does not cover all situations. In the early 70's, Dr. Kelly's wife was exposed to toxic paint fumes and developed severe chronic fatigue and almost died. The vegetarian diet and supplements that he used to cure his cancer failed to restore her health. In desperation, he began feeding his wife a broth made from raw ground meat. She made a swift and dramatic recovery. Doctor Kelly learned that a healthy diet for some people (vegetarianism) was a formula for disaster for others.

In the late 70's he became the first researcher to use the autonomic nervous system as the foundation for classifying people into metabolic categories or metabolic types, each with its own comprehensive nutritional protocol. This metabolic typing approach was responsible for reversing some 35,000 cancer patients. Doctor Kelly was fortunate to have an able assistant, William Wolcott, who worked with Dr. Kelly for fifteen years. Wolcott was able to integrate Dr. Kelly's work with the important research of the psychologist, George Watson. Watson discovered the oxidative (combustion of foods) system, which he successfully used to reverse many psychiatric problems that failed to respond to conventional medicine. The combined concepts offer cancer patients and their caregivers a rational dietary approach without a steep learning curve.

Dominance factor Any given nutrient will affect different people in different ways. How a given nutrient affects someone depends on the dominance factor of a particular metabolic type. The dominant system refers to the autonomic nervous and the oxidative systems. The autonomic nervous system (ANS) takes care of the peripheral areas of the body and is comprised of two parts: sympathetic and parasympathetic. This system helps maintain internal balance within the body by first perceiving the internal environment then modulating it by stimulating or inhibiting functions (chemical reactions, temperature changes, heart rate, muscle tone, rate of breathing, elimination and detoxification). The ANS, which is involuntary, that is, it works automatically via the lymphatic and circulatory systems and main organs: liver, gall bladder, spleen, stomach, pancreas, lungs, heart, adrenals, kidney, thyroid, parathyroid, thymus and intestines. Furthermore, the ANS helps regulate body function by varying blood flow (changing the diameter of the transporting vessels and heart rate). In essence, the ANS functions like an efficient dispatcher guaranteeing a smooth operation. When an imbalance occurs in the ANS, function shifts toward one or both of major divisions: the sympathetic or parasympathetic. Clinical symptoms reported by patients represent actual "normal" functions that have become exaggerated or suppressed. A cluster of symptoms (dry mouth, constipation, rapid heart rate, high blood pressure, poor digestion, dilated pupils) that reflect an increase activity of the sympathetic nervous system would be classified as sympathetic dominant. Likewise a cluster of symptoms (diarrhea, low blood pressure, chronic fatigue, irregular heart beat) that reflect an increase activity of the parasympathetic nervous system would be classified as parasympathetic dominant.

The other major component of metabolic typing is the oxidative system, which relates to the speed at which tissues of the body convert food to energy. As a result of his research on biological oxidation and metabolic individuality, Dr. George Watson, PhD., a full professor at the University of Southern California, discovered psychochemical states and their relationship to personality disorders. Doctor Watson was able to reverse such maladies as anxiety, depression and paranoid delusions by correcting oxidative imbalances. Watson was also able to induce psychiatric symptoms in normal people by restricting their diet in fats and protein. Patients deprived of daily fats and protein exhibited a wide range of symptoms from social withdrawal, anxiety and depression to violent and psychotic behavior.

Watson discovered that when the pH (acid/base balance) of venous blood deviated from the norm 4.76 it directly affected the body's ability to absorb and utilize enzymes and trace nutrients. People whose pH was below the ideal of 4.76 where classified as acidic (fast-oxidizers) and those above alkaline (slow-oxidizers). Acidic individuals, who were fast-oxidizers, required calcium to help rebalance their pH while others who were alkaline and slow-oxidizers required potassium, magnesium and manganese to regain homeostasis or normalization. Clinically, Watson discovered that fast-oxidizers exhibited many of the characteristics of functional hypoglycemia while slow-oxidizers functioned as diabetics.

Two (or more) people can have the same adverse symptom or health problem for opposite biochemical reasons. For example, if a person had leg cramps and was metabolically typed as a *Fast-Oxidizer (acidic)* an *increase* in calcium and a *decrease* in potassium would be indicated. However, in a *Slow-Oxidative Dominant* type *(alkaline)*, a *decrease* in calcium and an *increase* in potassium would be indicated.

Foods in themselves are not acidifying or alkalinizing to the body. Whether a food has an acid or an alkaline effect on the body depends not on its ash, but rather on the dominance factor in the metabolic type, i.e., on what system is most strongly affected by the foods. For example, if a high potassium food like a fruit or a vegetable that burns to an alkaline ash in the body is given to a *Parasympathetic Dominant (alkaline)* it will cause a shift toward alkalinity and hypoactive characteristics by increasing parasympathetic activity (slowed heart rate, increased digestion, decreased perspiration, increased salivation, increased secretion of digestive enzymes, increased peristaltic waves of the intestines, etc.).

On the other hand, in a *Fast-Oxidative Dominant (acidic)*, a high potassium food will speed food combustion, increase acidity, enhance hypoglycemic symptoms, and the parasympathetic part of the nervous system will be stimulated in an attempt to restore balance.

A sympathetic autonomic dominant tends to be a "class A" type personality — aggressive, hyperactive, competitive, and acidic in nature. If a sympathetic dominant (acid) is a slow-oxidizer (alkaline) the usual sympathetic personality may be totally altered by a diet high in protein and fat: hyperactive characteristics may be replaced by hypoactive tendencies; and an acid nature by a more alkaline one; aggression may be replaced with apathy, and so on. A diet high in protein and fat will further slow food combustion, increase alkalinity and lower energy levels. This serves to explain how a sympathetic type could experience depression, when in fact the lack of the experience of depression is usually a hallmark of sympathetic influence.

On the other hand, a sympathetic type that happens to be a fast-oxidative dominant would tend to have an ultra "class A" personality consuming a vegetarian type diet. Such behavior could easily be mistaken for sympathetic dominance, and vice versa. This exemplifies beautifully the danger of the "symptom treatment" approach to nutrition. Plain and simple, all class A personalities are not alike. Treating them all the same may help some of them, but it can also make others worse than before! For example, fruit tends to calm a sympathetic autonomic dominant, but tends to increase excitability in the fast-oxidative dominant. (see chart on Variable pH Effect of Foods–Page 172)

Balance and efficiency are intimately interrelated; equally connected are imbalance and inefficiency. For example, an imbalance in the nervous system may give rise to inefficiency in the function of an organ; restoring balance to the nervous system may result in the improvement of efficiency in the disturbed organ. However, it is also true that inefficiency in a gland, e.g., the adrenal glands, may give rise to an imbalance in the autonomic nervous system. Using medications to treat the clinical symptoms only serves to mask the problem while the underlying imbalance worsens.

EATING BEFORE BED

To eat or not to eat that is the question or at least part of the question. The other part concerns what to eat!

Certain metabolic types (parasympathetic or fast-oxidizers) may need to eat before going to bed. If these types don't eat, they usually experience difficulty falling asleep, and if they do fall asleep they will invariably awaken in the middle of the night. Usually, their ideal fuel mixture is a snack that contains a mix of protein and fat. A high carbohydrate snack may help some, but is usually not sufficient to carry them through the night. In these metabolic types, a high carbohydrate snack will actually be stimulating (by increasing the oxidation rate and energy) and thus, prevent sleep.

Other metabolic types (sympathetic and slow-oxidizers) generally don't do well eating before bed. They often complain that when they eat before going to bed, food feels like a rock in their stomachs. If they do eat a bedtime snack, they do best eating food high in carbohydrates with just a little protein and fat, like a small bowl of cereal with milk or some fruit and yogurt.

Salt Parasympathetic and slow-oxidizers tend to do better including high sodium foods and some salt in their diets to help balance body chemistry. But, in the sympathetic and fast-oxidizers, salt often has too strong of a stimulating effect on the adrenals and if eaten around bedtime may contribute to insomnia.

Calcium In the autonomic sympathetic dominant, calcium usually acts as a stimulant by innervating the sympathetic system. Thus, in the sympathetic dominant, calcium is not recommended before bed. However, in the extreme parasympathetic dominant that awakens in the night with hunger pains, calcium may help diminish the appetite by restoring autonomic balance. In this type, calcium before bed may help prevent the body chemistry from going too parasympathetic during the night.

In the fast-oxidative dominant, calcium tends to have a sedating, calming effect by slowing down the rate of oxidation. When the oxidation rate gets too fast, carbohydrates are "burned" too quickly. The result is that one also runs out of fuel too quickly as well. When this occurs at night, insomnia may result. Calcium before bed for the fast-oxidizer may help prevent this from occurring.

Magnesium In the autonomic sympathetic dominant, magnesium acts as a natural tranquilizer by inhibiting the influence of the sympathetic system (quite the adrenal gland function). In the sympathetic insomniac characterized by racing thoughts or an inability to shut the mind off when trying to sleep, magnesium has been found to be an excellent bedtime supplement.

Potassium Whereas calcium is the mineral which acts as the major stimulator of the sympathetic system, potassium is considered the major innervater of the parasympathetic system. In the sympathetic dominant, magnesium and potassium work well together, producing a calming, sedating influence.

On the other hand, in the fast-oxidizer, potassium tends to have a stimulating effect. The result may be a strong increase in appetite.

Thymus While the sympathetic system is responsible for energy, motivation, get-up-and-go, the parasympathetic system controls immune function, digestion and all repairing/rebuilding activity. Thus, it is the parasympathetic system, which normally dominates during sleep. Certain glands are related to the sympathetic system while others are related to the parasympathetic system. The thymus is considered to be the major "parasympathetisizing" gland of the endocrine system. Stimulation and support of the thymus has been observed to increase parasympathetic tone, particularly when used along with magnesium and potassium.

Other parasympathetic glandulars, singularly or in formulas, may be used along with thymus for a stronger parasympathetisizing influence.

Tryptophan Taken before bed this amino acid encourages sleep, particularly when combined with a carbohydrate. Ingestion of carbohydrates (starchy and sweet foods) stimulates insulin release, which aids tryptophan's journey to the brain and conversion to the sedating neurotransmitter, serotonin. It appears to be most effective for parasympathetic dominant types, but has not been found to be of much help in other metabolic types with insomnia.

Adrenal In rare instances, insomnia may be related to adrenal insufficiency. This type of insomnia is characterized by falling asleep, only to "jerk" awake 20-30 minutes later. It may be accompanied by feelings of panic and/or a racing heart. Some adrenal support along with other nutritional support of the sympathetic system may prove helpful. Often a bedtime snack including meat or poultry is often of benefit. With adrenal insufficiency, use of an adaptogen like Rhodiola rosea found in the product Optygen™ has proven very effective.

Herbs Herbs used in tea or capsule form may help support and balance body chemistry. Herbs are almost always better when taken in combination as opposed to individually. They are available in most health food store's prepackaged blends.

Valerian root, wild lettuce, blue vervain, catnip, blue violet, passion flower, and scullcap are best for sympathetics. Comfrey root, horsetail (shavegrass), oat straw, lobelia, chamomile and dandelion may be more suited to parasympathetics.

Additional information on metabolic typing is available at Dr. Harold Kristal's web site: *http://www.ernaehrungstyp.de/library.html*

HISTORY OF METABOLIC TYPING

1930-1940 Francis Pottenger, MD pioneer in nutritional science

Royal Lee, DDS pioneer in nutritional science

Both men recognized that people had unique dietary requirements and discovered that the autonomic nervous system holds important clues to predict what types of foods and nutrients people need.

1960-1970 William Donald Kelly, DDS biologist, chemist, biochemist and pioneer in nutritional science

- Regarded as the "father of metabolic typing"
- *Mid-1960's* Kelly developed pancreatic cancer — and was given a few months to live. He put together an eclectic approach using diet, vitamins, minerals, enzymes and detoxification techniques and Kelly reversed his pancreatic cancer.
- *Early 70's* Kelly's wife was exposed to toxic paint fumes and developed severe chronic

fatigue and almost died. His standard vegetarian diet, and supplements failed to restore her health. In desperation, he began feeding his wife meat. She made a swift and dramatic recovery. Kelly learned that a healthy diet for some people (vegetarianism) was a formula for disaster for others.

- *Late 70's* He was the first researcher to use the ANS as the foundation for classifying people into metabolic categories or metabolic types, each with its own comprehensive nutritional protocol.

1981 George Watson, Ph.D. Clinical psychologist. Author of *Nutrition and Your Mind*. Pioneer in nutritional science. Watson discovered that certain nutrients intensified adverse emotional states in some patients, while in others, the same nutrients could alleviate emotional problems. He discovered a distinct correlation between people's psychological and emotional characteristics and the rate at which their cells convert nutrients into energy. Watson used foods and nutrients to balance the patient's cellular oxidation rates and resolve their emotional problems.

1990's William L. Wolcott World's leading authority on metabolic typing. Author of *Metabolic Typing Diet* Wolcott developed a system for detecting autonomic dominance versus oxidative dominance. "The Dominance Factor"

Characteristics Associated with

SYMPATHETIC DOMINANCE VS PARASYMPATHETIC DOMINANCE

Physical Tendencies	Physical Tendencies
▪ indigestion	▪ diarrhea
▪ heartburn	▪ allergies
▪ insomnia	▪ irregular heartbeat
▪ hypertension	▪ low blood sugar
▪ high blood pressure	▪ chronic fatigue
▪ predisposed to infection	▪ cold sores
▪ low appetite	▪ excessive appetite
▪ angular facial structure	▪ round face and skull
▪ tendency to be tall	▪ shorter, wider build

Psychological/Behavioral Tendencies	Psychological/Behavioral Tendencies
▪ excellent concentration	▪ lethargy
▪ highly motivated	▪ procrastination
▪ cool emotionally	▪ slow to anger
▪ irritable	▪ deliberate, cautious
▪ hyperactive	▪ warm emotionally
▪ socially withdrawn	▪ socially outgoing

The sympathetic part of the nervous system is like a car's gas pedal. In emergency situations the heart beats quickly, the mouth becomes dry, the pupils dilate, digestion slows, and perspiration increases. The parasympathetic part of the nervous system functions like the car's breaks. It becomes activated during mealtime with increased salivation, increased flow of digestive juices, increased movement of the intestine, pupils constrict, slowed heart rate and decreased perspiration. Imbalance of this system will directly affect the acid-base balance, and directly influence cancer. The more acid one becomes, the lower the oxygen level and the more ideal the condition to support cancer growth. Dietary selection is extremely important in helping to balance these two parts of the nervous system. Using the metabolic typing approach is a more intelligent way to assist restoring one's health in the shortest period of time.

"One of the fundamental problems with nutritional science is that it lacks a logical system of reference points a system with enough flexibility to accommodate all the biological diversity among people. The only reference points it has are 'normal ranges', fixed values that are supposed to represent optimal, healthy levels of nutrients. These so-called 'normal ranges' are actually just averages of nutrient levels typically found in the population. The general population is a heterogeneous mix of all different kinds of metabolic types. Roger Williams, Ph.D. (University Texas 1930's) points out, it's not unusual to find as much as a one hundred fold difference in nutrient level requirements from one person to the next."

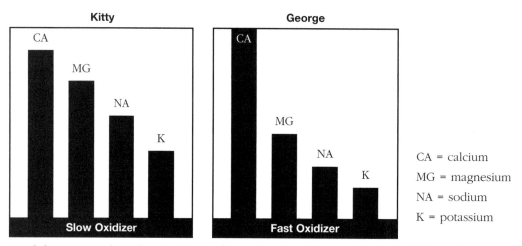

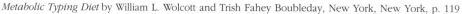

Metabolic Typing Diet by William L. Wolcott and Trish Fahey Boubleday, New York, New York, p. 119

The above hair analysis chart shows two people with identical nutrient excesses and deficiencies. Thus they would appear to require the same kind of nutritional protocol. But in reality, these people require opposite nutritional protocols. As a slow oxidizer, Kitty resolved her chronic health problems with a high-potassium/low calcium protocol. And as a fast oxidizer, George was able to resolve his problems with a low potassium/high-calcium protocol. This shows why a tissue level substance (hair) is not a reliable indicator of cellular nutrient requirements and why metabolic typing provides a crucial frame of reference for interpreting nutrient levels found in the body and in turn establishing correct nutritional protocols. Because Kitty was a slow-oxidizer, we know her cellular calcium levels are high and we know her tissue levels are high from the hair analysis. Thus we know she has a quantitative excess of calcium. But because George is a fast-oxidizer, we know his cellular calcium levels are low. And because his hair tissue levels are high, he has a qualitative insufficiency, meaning that there is enough calcium present in his body, but qualitatively, it is neither where it should be (in the cells) nor is it being used properly.

Reading Metabolic Typing Diet provides an understanding of why the same diet cannot be prescribed to all patients. Eating quality food or nutritional supplements that are inappropriate for the metabolic type can stimulate cancer growth.

VITAMINS, MINERALS BENEFICIAL TO SYMPATHETIC DOMINANCE

The following nutrients work by stimulating the parasympathetic nervous system:

Slow Oxidizers	
■ B2 Riboflavin	■ Inositol
■ B 3 Niacin	■ Folic acid
■ B6 Pyridoxine	■ Magnesium
■ Betaine	■ Para-amino Benzoic acid
■ Biotin	■ Potassium
■ Choline	■ Zinc

VITAMINS, MINERALS BENEFICIAL TO PARASYMPATHETIC DOMINANCE

The following nutrients work by stimulating the sympathetic nervous system:

Fast Oxidizers	
■ B1 Thiamine	■ B4 Antiparalysis factor
■ B5 Pantothenic acid	■ B12 Cobalamin
■ Calcium	■ Phosphorous
■ Arginine	■ Boron

Variable pH Effect of Foods

AUTONOMIC-DOMINANT TYPE vs OXIDATIVE-DOMINANT TYPE

Vegetables	Parasympathetic (alk) alkalinize Sympathetic (acid) alkalinize	Fat oxidizer (acidic) acidify Slow oxidizer (alkaline) acidify
Meats	Sympathetic (acidic) acidify Parasympathetic (alk) acidify	Slow oxidizer (alkaline) alkalinize Fast oxidizer (acidic) alkalinize

One important way in which foods or nutrients affect health is by influencing the body's acid/alkaline balance. Changes in pH are more often due to the effect of foods on the fundamental homeostatic controls, than on the pH of the foods' ash. *It is not the food or nutrient itself that determines acid or alkaline effects in the body, but the dominant system influenced by that food that is behind it all and ultimately determines the acid/alkaline result and other reactions to nutrients.*

The chart above depicts the effects of specific food groups on autonomic and oxidative types. Ingestion of vegetables by a parasympathetic dominant who is already alkaline will make them more alkaline and worsen their condition. A sympathetic dominant, who is acidic, will benefit eating a vegetarian type diet. On the other hand, when a fast-oxidizer (already acidic) consumes vegetables, a more acidic condition results with a worsening of symptoms. Since a slow-oxidizer is alkaline, they will benefit from eating vegetables; high carbohydrate foods like vegetables will also speed up the combustion rate of food. Meats given to a sympathetic dominant person will worsen their condition by making them more acid. A parasympathetic dominant, which is alkaline, however, will benefit by eating meat because their nervous system will balance out. Meat consumed by a slow-oxidizer who is already alkaline will also witness a worsening of symptoms where as a fast-oxidizer will benefit by eating meat because it will slow the combustion rate of the food.

Contrary to conventional wisdom, foods and nutrients have no fixed or inherent acid/alkaline qualities. The very same food, meat for example, will produce an alkaline shift in an oxidative type and produce an opposite (acidic) shift in an autonomic type.

Acid/Alkaline Balance Two of the seven factors that cancer patients must focus on are known to influence pH. Since it is beyond the scope of this book, the other five factors will not be discussed.

- ***Autonomic Nervous System:*** Sympathetic (acid), Parasympathetic (alkaline)
- ***Oxidative:*** Fast oxidizer (acid), slow oxidizer (alkaline)
- Catabolic/anabolic system
- Electrolyte/fluid balance

- Endocrine regulation (pituitary, thyroid, parathyroid, adrenal, gonads)
- Respiration
- Acid/alkaline ash foods

Thyroid-Suppressing Foods Thiocyanates, which are present in raw broccoli, Brussel sprouts, cabbage, cauliflower, kale, mustard greens, rutabaga and watercress, block the production of thyroid hormone.

Foods high in gluten Wheat (and most grains), oats, rye and all by-products should be avoided by the Group II parasympathetic metabolic type. The wheat makes the patient more acidic and more parasympathetic. Also gluten is hard to digest and is linked to allergies, celiac disease (sprue), mental illness, indigestion and yeast overgrowth. Soaking and fermentation renders such protein more digestible. Sourdough, millet and sprouted breads (Manna, Ezekiel) are preferable.

Metabolic Type	Diet	Metabolic Imbalance
Protein Type 70% Proteins and fats 30% Carbohydrates	high protein — 40% heavy, fatty, high purine proteins high fats and oils — 30% low carbohydrates	fast oxidizer or parasympathetic dominent
Carbohydrate Type 60% Carbohydrates 40% Proteins and fats	low protein light, lean, low purine proteins low fats and oils — 30% high carbohydrates	slow oxidizer or sympathetic dominent
Mixed Type 50% Proteins and fats 50% Carbohydrates	mixture of high-fat, high-purine proteins and low-fat, low-purine proteins requires relatively equal ratios of proteins, fats and carbohydrates	neither fast nor slow oxidizer neither parasympathetic or sympathetic dominent

Regardless of what metabolic type one is classified, close scrutiny must be paid to the glycemic index of food. The primary concern in cancer patients is to select foods that will not markedly raise the blood sugar. This process is expedited by use of the glycemic index, which ranks foods in their ability to increase the blood sugar within two to three hours after eating. Foods with a high glycemic index stimulate rapid insulin production, which enhances fat deposits and interferes with conversion of fat into energy. Care must also be taken not to consume large amounts of protein, which will interfere with the use of pancreatic enzymes that are designed to digest the outer protein covering of cancer cells. This judicious process will result in *weight loss*, which alarms most oncologists not familiar with nutritional approaches to reversing cancer. It may require six months before the body's weight stabilizes. The ultimate goal is to starve the cancer while simultaneously employing various technology and nutrients to destroy the cancer and then permit healing and regeneration.

The closer the program is followed the faster resolution is realized. In my wife's case, the integrated therapies resulted in total resolution that was confirmed by the CA 125 tumor marker of 2.2 and negative CAT Scan of the abdominal region. The approach put forth in this book is comprehensive. The best diagnostic medical records available have documented the results. The three general metabolic categories provide an effective starting point for customizing the diet.

GLYCEMIC INDEX CHART — HIGH/MEDIUM GLYCEMIC INDEX FOODS

Sugar	Grains	Vegetables
110 maltose, beer alcohol	91 instant rice	101 parsnip
100 glucose	90 puffed rice	88 potato (baked)
95 glucose and sports drinks	89 Rice Chex	86 potato (instant mashed)
83 jelly beans	85 pretzels	78 French fries
73 life savers	82 Rice Krispies	78 pumpkin
70 jams	80 Corn Flakes	77 corn chips
68 soft drinks	80 rice cakes	75 rutabaga
65 corn syrup	75 wheat cereals	68 cornmeal
65 sucrose (table sugar)	75 graham crackers	66 beets
61 honey	74 Cheerios	59 corn
51 chocolate	72 bagel	58 popcorn
Fruits	72 whole-wheat bread	56 sweet potato
103 dates	72 white bread	53 yam
75 watermellons	72 saltine crackers	51 carrot
68 cantaloupe	71 millet	51 green peas
67 pineapple	70 pancakes	51 potato chips
66 raisins	69 Rye-Krisp	
62 bananas	67 Shredded Wheat	
60 apricots	67 Grape Nuts	
55 mango	67 couscous	
52 kiwi	66 brown rice	
Dairy	66 Cream of Wheat	
61 ice cream	67 brown rice pasta	
52 ice cream (low-fat)	66 Muesli	
	59 sweet corn	
	59 pastry	
	53 oatmeal (instant)	
	51 buckwheat	
	51 All-Bran	
	50 rye bread	

GLYCEMIC INDEX CHART — LOW GLYCEMIC INDEX FOODS

Sugar	Grains	Vegetables
43 lactose	49 oatmeal (whole grain)	48 dried peas
20 fructose	49 wheat bran	42 pinto beans
Fruits	47 bulgur	40 baked beans (canned)
46 orange juice	46 whole-wheat pasta	38 tomato soup
45 grapes	42 whole-wheat spaghetti	38 navy beans
41 apple juice	34 rye	36 chick peas
40 oranges	22 barley	36 lima beans
38 apples	19 rice bran	30 black-eyed peas
36 pears	**Fruits**	32 split peas
32 strawberries	36 flavored yogurt	30 black beans
30 bananas (unripe)	30 butter	29 kidney beans
29 peaches		29 lentiles
26 grapefruit		23 dried peas
25 plums		15 soy beans
23 cherries		14 green vegetables

METABOLIC DIET TYPING QUESTIONNAIRE

Please check off those main characteristics that best apply to you and circle the dot of those characteristics that directly apply. For a more in depth questionnaire, please refer to the book Metabolic Typing Diet (page 135) by William L. Wolcott.

Group I — Slow-Oxidizer/Sympathetic Dominant

☐ *Relatively weak appetite*
- Eating a little food goes a long way.
- Small meals tend to satisfy hunger.
- Satisfies with one or two meals and several smaller snacks.
- Food does not play a prominent role in conscious daily awareness.

☐ *High tolerance for sweets*
- Handle sweets pretty well.
- Tendency to eat sweets when ever hungry or need an energy boost.
- Tendency to overdo eating sweets.

☐ *Problems with weight management*
- Tendency to be lean during adolescence.
- Tendency to be overweight with sweet-snacking.
- Can go long periods between eating.

☐ *Type-A personality*

- Tendency to be aggressive, goal-oriented, highly motivated workaholic.

- Can be abrupt, appear cool and aloof and quick to anger.

- Energy tends to come in spurts — physical stamina is relatively limited.

- Concentration tends to be excellent.

- Often times think they do not have time to eat.

☐ *Variable energy pattern*

- Lower steadier energy without the peaks and valleys.

☐ *Caffeine dependency*

- Depend on having caffeine through the day.

- Overuse weakens appetite or worsens dietary habits.

- Feel as though cannot live without caffeine.

METABOLIC DIET TYPING QUESTIONNAIRE

Please check off those main characteristics that best apply to you and circle the dot of those characteristics that directly apply.

Group II — Fast-Oxidizer/Parasympathetic Dominant

☐ *Strong appetite*

- Ravenously hungry a great deal of the time.

- Feel the need to eat frequently.

- Hard time feeling satisfied after eating meals or snacks.

- Tendency to overeat sometimes.

☐ *Cravings for fatty, salty foods*

- Gravitate toward rich, fatty, salty foods like sausage, pizza and roasted and salted nuts.

☐ *Crave sugar*

- Eating too many carbohydrates causes a craving for sugar.

- Craving for sugar increases with increased consumption of sugar.

- Eating sugar causes a drop in energy, feel nervous and jittery.

☐ *Failure with weight loss*

- Eating a low-calorie diet causes weight to increase or stay the same.

- Starvation diets cause weight gain or no change.

☐ *Feelings of fatigue, anxiety or nervousness*

- Feel either lethargy or energized.

- Experience low energy and prone to feel apathetic, depressed, listless and sleepy.

- Feel wired or edgy but internally feel exhausted.

- Feelings of anxiousness, nervousness and jitteriness improve with eating.

METABOLIC DIET TYPING QUESTIONNAIRE

Please check off those main characteristics that best apply to you and circle the dot of those characteristics that directly apply.

Group III — Mixed Oxidizer

☐ *Variable appetite*

- Tends to have an average appetite.
- Tends to feel hungry at mealtime but typically does not get hungry at other times.
- Appetite tends to vacillate — sometimes feel ravenous while other times not hungry even to the point of skipping meals.

☐ *Craving for sweets and carbohydrates*

- Typically does not get cravings.

☐ *Weight control*

- Tends to do well with the widest range of foods.
- Less of a problem with weight.
- Can easily develop a weight problem with restricted diets.

☐ *Fatigue, anxiety and nervousness*

- Experiences fatigue, lethargy or depression when following a restricted diet.
- Less likely to develop medical problems.

FOOD PREFERENCES AND REACTIONS FOR FAST-AND SLOW-OXIDIZERS

Fast-Oxidizers	Slow-Oxidizers
grapefruit juice tastes too sour	likes grapefruit juice
likes potatoes	
mustard tastes and smells too shard	likes mustard
likes avacados, olives, mayonaise	finds avacados too fatty
likes salty foods	craves sweet and sour foods
sweet foods often taste too sweet	sweets increase appetite
likes bacon with meats	likes onions with meat
coffee causes jitteryness	likes coffee
requires breakfast	doesn't want breakfast
feels weak if doesn't eat every 2-3 hours	when nauseous, sweet and sour foods help
likes well-done roast beef	gets thirsty and requires a lot of water

FOODS TO AVOID ACCORDING TO YOUR BLOOD TYPE

Blood Type A	Blood Type B	Blood Type AB	Blood Type O
blackberries	bitter pear melons	blackberries	blackberries
brown trout	black-eyed peas	black-eyed peas	chocolate
clams	castor beans	brown trout	cocoa
cornflakes	chicken	clams	French mushrooms (amanita muscaria)
French mushrooms (hygrophorus hypothejus)	chocolate	cocoa	halibut
halibut	cocoa	cornflakes	flounder
flounder	French mushrooms (hygrophorus hypothejus, morasmius orcodes)	French mushrooms (hygrophorus hypothejus)	sole
lima beans	pomegranates	halibut	sunflower seeds
snow white mushrooms	salmon	flounder	
sole	sesame	lima beans	
soybean sprouts	sunflower seeds	pomegranates	
string beans	soybeans	salmon	
tore beans	tuna	sesame	
		snow white mushrooms	
		sole	
		soybeans	
		soybean sprouts	
		string beans	
		sunflower seeds	
		tuna	

GROUP I AND II DIETS: pHs OF THE METABOLIC TYPES

Acid (-)	Alkaline (+)
fast-oxidizer	slow-oxidizer
sympathetic	parasympathetic

DIET GROUPING OF THE METABOLIC TYPES

Group I	Group II
slow-oxidizer	fast-oxidizer
sympathetic	parasympathetic

DIETS OF THE GROUP I AND II METABOLIC TYPES

Group I	Group II
slow-oxidizer	fast-oxidizer
sympathetic	parasympathetic
lower protein and fats	higher protein and fats
higher complex carbs	lower complex carbs

Fast and slow-oxidizers can often be identified by their food preferences and reactions. Refer to the table on page 177 to help make the distinction.

- Dietary lectins — protein substances that are found in small quantities in about thirty percent of our foods. Lectins are blood-type specific, i.e., they will only cause negative effects in people with specific blood types.
- Cooking and digestion inhibit the activity of lectins to some extent, however many find their way into the bloodstream where they act as antigens (foreign substances).
- Certain lectins bind to the surfaces of specific blood cell types (A, B, O or AB).
- Lectins frequently cause agglutination (clumping) and subsequent lysing (destruction) of blood cells.

GROUP I FOODS: SLOW-OXIDIZER AND SYMPATHETIC

PROTEINS			CARBOHYDRATES			FATS
Meat	**Seafood**	**Dairy**	**Grains**	**Vegetables**	**Fruits**	**Oils/Nuts**
Eat light meats and avoid dark meat	Eat white fish and shellfish only	Limited use of low or non-fat only	All are OK (except oats) Include	Emphasize the following	All are OK Include	Use sparingly
poultry breast	catfish	yogurt	amaranth	beet	apples	almonds
lean pork	cod	cottage cheese	barley	broccoli	berries	almond butter
Minimize	flounder	cheese	buckwheat	brussel sprouts	cherries	olive oil
oats	haddock	milk	millet	cabbage	citrus	**Moderately**
salty foods	perch	**Misc.**	quinoa	cucumber	grapes	coconut oil
fatty foods	scrod	eggs	brown rice	eggplant	melons	sesame oil
organ meat	sole		rye	garlic	peaches	
red meat	trout		wheat	leafy green	pineapple	
butter	tuna (white)		**Very Best**	lettuce	plum	
avocado	crab		grass juices	onions		
artichoke	crayfish		barley/wheat	peppers		
asparagus	lobster			potatos		
carrots	shrimp			sprouts		
cauliflower				soft squash		
olives				tomatoes		
peas/beans				turnips		
spinach				yams		
				zucchini		

- Lectins can interfere with digestion and absorption and cause a host of other problems: nutrient deficiencies, food allergies, inflammatory bowel disease, diabetes mellitus, rheumatoid arthritis, psoriasis, infertility, intestinal gas, immune deficiencies, fatigue, headaches, achiness, diarrhea, irritability and anemia.
- Cancer patients are advised to follow the recommendations as closely as possible.

Group I metabolic types require less protein and fats. Their protein must be in the form of lighter meats like white-meat chicken and turkey and less oily fishes primarily white fish. (Complex carbohydrates provide the slow-oxidizing person the quick-burning fuel needed to speed up their oxidation rate and help put on the breaks to slow down the sympathetic nervous system.) Too much protein and fats will suppress the slow-oxidative type by decreasing their metabolism and further fuel their sympathetic characteristics. The Group I diet is well suited to vegetarians. The Group I vegetarians need to consume a higher proportion of legumes (peas, beans, peanuts, lentils) to provide adequate quantities of protein.

Group II metabolic types require much more protein and fat than Group I types. Proteins and fats slow down the oxidation process (combustion of food for energy) of the Group II person. The energy generated is slower and more even. Since the Group II type is parasympathetic and has a tendency to be sluggish, proteins and fats will stimulate the sympathetic part of the nervous system and increase their energy. Overall the Group II's do better consuming darker meats (red meat, dark-chicken and poultry) and oilier fish (salmon, sardines, herring and dark tuna) and proteins that are higher in purines (organ meats, sardines, anchovies, fish eggs) and moderately high in lentils. The purines are nitrogen-based proteins that deliver more energy. *This group must avoid wheat and wheat products because they make fast-oxidizers more acid and parasympathetics much more alkaline.* Because fruit is a carbohydrate it should be a small part of the diet. It is extremely difficult for Group II's to be vegetarians. Vegetarians can do better if they modify their diet to include eggs, dairy products and fish.

GROUP II FOODS: FAST-OXIDIZER AND PARASYMPATHETIC

PROTEINS			CARBOHYDRATES			FATS
Meat	**Seafood**	**Dairy**	**Grains**	**Vegetables**	**Fruits**	**Oils/Nuts**
All are OK emphasize dark meats	All are OK emphasize oily fish	All whole milk is OK (cow, goat, sheep)	Most are OK (except wheat)	Only have the following	Only have the following	All oils, nuts and seeds are OK, including
poultry dark	salmon	yogurt	amaranth	artichoke	apples (tart)	butter
liver/kidneys	sardines	cottage cheese	buckwheat	asparagus	Granny Smith	nut butters
red meat	mackerel	cheese	corn	avocado	Pippins	**Oils**
Minimize	herring	cream	millet	carrots	pears (firm)	coconut
wheat and all by-products	tuna (dark)	milk	oats	cauliflower	Bosc	olive
white rice	anchovies	**Misc.**	quinoa	celery	D'Anjou	sesame
broccoli	caviar/roe	algae	rice (brown)	green beans	banana (firm)	**Nuts/Seeds**
potatoes	crab	eggs	rye	jicama	**Moderately**	walnuts
mustard greens	shrimp	tempeh		mushrooms	apricots	pecans
soft squashes	oysters	tofu		olives	berries	cashews
tomatoes	shellfish	beans		peas	plums	almonds
zucchini		lentils		spinach		brazils
citrus fruit				winter squash		pumpkin
grapes				**Moderately**		sunflower
fruit juice				chard		
vinegar				green salad		
				kale		

GROUP I MENU PLAN: SUGGESTED MENUS ONLY

	Breakfast	Lunch	Dinner
Monday	yogurt (low-fat) fruit almonds	chicken sandwich green salad	grilled sole steamed greens baked potato
Tuesday	wheat (or corn) flakes low-fat milk whole wheat toast	turkey burger coleslaw mixed vegetables	chicken noodle soup pasta (with marinara)
Wednesday	poached eggs whole wheat toast	tuna salad clam chowder	chicken curry brown rice cucumber salad
Thursday	cottage cheese (low-fat), fruit almonds	chicken salad French onion soup	leek and potato soup eggplant parmesan green salad
Friday	cream of wheat milk (low-fat) fruit	chicken burrito chips (baked) and salsa	broiled halibut brussels sprouts green salad
Saturday	whole wheat waffles fruit turkey bacon	egg salad sandwich vegetable soup	chicken risotto steamed greens
Sunday	soft boiled eggs chicken sausage whole wheat toast	tuna salad wheat crackers	turkey breast potatoes steamed broccoli

Snacks The Group I Metabolic Types generally do not require much in the way of snacks. However, if snacks are desired, they should be selected from the same suggested foods as the primary meals. Suggested snacks include:

- Fruit
- Almonds
- Yogurt or cottage cheese (low-fat)
- Whole wheat (or other whole grain) crackers with low-fat cheese or almond butter

GROUP II MENU PLAN: SUGGESTED MENUS ONLY

	Breakfast	Lunch	Dinner
Monday	yogurt (whole milk) sandwich non-wheat	vegetable soup	bacon and avocado meatloaf green beans
Tuesday	scrambled eggs turkey bacon	caesar salad lentil soup	salmon casserole steamed artichokes grated carrot salad
Wednesday	oatmeal whey powder banana	chicken sandwich carrot and celery sticks, olives	baked salmon steamed cauliflower spinach salad
Thursday	soft-boiled eggs bacon toast (non-wheat)	greek salad bean soup	roast chicken sauteed mushrooms asparagus
Friday	cottage cheese (whole milk), cream of asparagus, blueberries, walnuts	corn on the cob kidney bean salad	hamburger patty sardines spinach salad
Saturday	buckwheat pancakes molasses turkey bacon	lamb chops steamed spinach or chard, sweet corn	miso soup sushi (brown rice)
Sunday	avocado and cheese omelet, toast (non-wheat), baked winter squash	mixed seafood casserole, quinoa, millet or brown rice	steak carrots and peas

Snacks The Group II Metabolic Types typically require snacks between meals, especially in the mid or late afternoon. The snacks should be protein and/or fat based; carbohydrates should not be eaten alone except, perhaps, an occasional piece of fruit.

Suggested snacks include:

- Olives
- Half an avocado
- Sardines or tuna (dark)
- Mixed nuts and seeds
- Banana with walnuts
- Half an apple with a piece of cheese

- Celery or carrot sticks with nut butter
- Yogurt or cottage cheese (full fat/whole milk)
- Rye or brown rice crackers with avocado, cheese or nut butter

"Have patience with all things, but chiefly have patience with yourself. Do not loose courage in considering your own imperfections but instantly set about remedying them — every day begin the task anew."

Saint Francis de Sales (1567-1622)

Section 7

TREATING THE PSYCHOLOGICAL
COMPONENT

PSYCHOLOGICAL COMPONENT

The two most traumatic events in my wife's life dealt with cancer. The first occurred in 1997 when she was diagnosed with breast cancer. The second was on December 9, 2002 when she was diagnosed with stage III ovarian cancer. The first episode instilled a level of fear beyond what she could ever imagine. The primary fear was the fear of dying. Overlaid on the uncontrollable feeling of fear was a dark cloud of depression. The psychological components of fear and depression caused both mental and physical paralysis. It was virtually impossible for her to get out of bed, shop, go to the beauty shop, talk to friends and family, and face life. This isolated lifestyle was filled with anxiety and daily crying spells that lasted four months. The turning point came when the decision to get post-surgical radiation therapy was made. Making this supreme decision dissipated most of the distress and the paralyzing fear of dying.

The cancer center, which provided the radiation treatment, also offered counseling as part of their comprehensive patient care program. The counseling sessions offered a venue for venting feelings of anxiety and fear, and re-establishing a more positive attitude about life and self worth. The therapy sessions proved to be a catalyst that hastened the emotional recovery.

There is nothing like experience to give one the confidence to face a similar traumatic situation. Learning of the presence of ovarian cancer was like a tsunami wave unleashing its fury on an unprotected coastline. The shock was devastating at first and reached a crescendo when the statistics and aggressiveness of ovarian cancer were understood. The fear, anxiety and crying episodes were there again but fewer shorter in duration and less severe. This time professional help was sought as soon as the surgical wounds healed and mobility was restored. A gifted patient of mine provided a unique form of therapy, which corrected energy blockages in the body. Her innate abilities coupled with the skills learned through training with Peruvian shamans were honed by incorporating the powerful Kathara Bio-Spiritual Healing System (*www.azuritepress.com*). Although esoteric, the results were spectacular. The feelings of heaviness in the chest and anxiety quickly dissipated allowing for a more normal daily schedule.

In my opinion, much of the fear and anxiety associated with cancer comes from the unknown and mysterious atmosphere cast by the medical establishment. The more people are kept in the dark about the underlying causes of cancer the greater the pervading fear and dread. And if the medical/pharmaceutical establishment controls the facilities and types of treatments, patients will never have options. In fact during the many conversations and consultations with the oncological surgeon, gynecologist, nurses and other medical personnel, never once was it ever suggested that alternative therapies are available and that we should explore them. The fear factor is heightened and perpetuated by the medical establishment's own ignorance and grim cancer statistics. The culmination of this fatalistic saga is the illusion that medicine has the gold standard for cancer treatment.

It is in the patient's best interest to read this book and explore alternative cancer support groups, Internet searches, alternative cancer consultants and alternative physicians. By understanding the nature of the cancer process the fear factor and anxiety level will diminish. By researching and taking an active part in the healing process patients become empowered. Following the traditional route of presenting the body to a physician for healing places one in the helpless victim mode mentality. Taking any positive steps toward healing are better than none. For some patients professional counseling will assist in helping to better cope with the realities of dealing with treatment, its side effects and its potential outcomes. Be willing to embrace the concept that what ever works is worth perusing.

Bach Flower Essences Dr. Edward Bach, MD in the early 1930's, developed an ingenious system of using energy patterns from wild flowers.

Theory: All chronic disease starts in the mind and emotions, unless obvious external factors are responsible.

Philosophy: The patient's mental/emotional condition will influence the course of recovery and affect the efficiency of medications. The mind and emotions play an important role in the processes of disease and its cure.

Initial Discovery: There are seven major personality types, which have their own specific intestinal flora. This indicates that intestinal floras not only mirror the physical health but also have an affinity for the personality type with its accompanying major mental/emotional tendencies.

False Assumption: Treating the seven specific intestinal flora with nosodes would resolve the patient's problem. The original treatment with nosodes (homeopathic preparations of actual pathogens) focused attention primarily on the physical factors as the primary cause and viewed the associated mental/emotional symptoms as secondary.

Bach's Research: Substantiated the fact that use of specific plants was capable of reversing the mental/emotional issues as well as reversing the associated pathogenic flora.

Objective: To strengthen the whole personality, including the body.

Healing Concept: His clinical observation determined that there were twelve healers or principal states of mind or personality tendencies:

- Fear and shyness: *(Mimulus)*
- Terror: *(Rock Rose)*
- Mental torture or worry: *(Agrimony)*
- Indecision: *(Scleranthus)*
- Indifference or bordem: *(Clematis)*
- Doubt or discouragement: *(Gentian)*
- Over concern for welfare of others: *(Chicory)*
- Weakness, cannot say no: *(Centaury)*
- Self-distrust: *(Cerato)*
- Impatience: *(Impatience)*
- Over enthusiasm: *(Vervain)*
- Pride or aloofness: *(Water Violet)*

Continued Research: Dr. Bach discovered twenty-six additional states of mind. The original twelve healers addressed the core personalities whereas the additional seven helpers focused on long-standing states of mental/emotional suffering that have become entrenched in the character as a whole and have begun to overshadow the true personality.

Seven Helper Essences:
- Hopelessness: *(Gorse)*s
- Despondency from overwork: *(Oak)*
- Self-centered, talkativeness: *(Heather)*
- Hard master onto oneself, with urge to inspire others: *(Rock Water)*
- Lack of motivation and incentive: *(Wild Oat)*
- Mental/emotional and physical weariness: *(Olive)*
- Domination of others: *(Vine)*

Nineteen Temporary States: Arise from circumstantial experiences of life. These 19 mental/emotional states can be part of the personality for prolonged periods of time but are not considered actual character traits.

- Fear of losing mental balance: *(Cherry Plum)*
- Vague fears and foreboding: *(Aspen)*
- Fear for others' welfare: *(Red Chestnut)*
- Mental fatigue: *(Hornbeam)*
- Longing for past happiness, nostalgia: *(Honeysuckle)*
- Feeling of powerlessness: *(Wild Rose)*
- Lack of mental tranquility: *(White Chestnut)*
- Depression and gloom: *(Mustard)*
- Immaturity of mind/emotions, failure to learn from mistakes: *(Chestnut Bud)*
- Vexations and jealousy: *(Holly)* Later added to helpers
- Easy impressionability: *(Walnut)*
- Shame or feelings of uncleanliness: *(Crab Apple)*
- Resentment and bitterness: *(Willow)*
- Sadness, grief and shock: *(Star of Bethlehem)*
- Despair and faithlessness: *(Sweet Chestnut)*
- Being overwhelmed: *(Elm)*
- Guilt and self-blame: *(Pine)*
- Low self-esteem: *(Larch)*
- Intolerance and criticism: *(Beech)*

Edward Bach's final system provides seven groups, which represent seven major areas of consciousness, where mental/emotional imbalances can occur. Each group, except for the Despondency or Despair, contains one or two of the basic type remedies. Bach discovered that his flower remedies *cured* the states of consciousness by more subtler and more finely tuned vibrations, which resulted from the delicate means of preparation.

For those who have fear:
- *Rock Rose* (core remedy): Terror
- *Mimulus* (core remedy): Fear of known things
- *Cherry Plum* (temporary state): Fear of losing mental control
- *Aspen* (temporary state): Fear of unknown
- *Red Chestnut* (temporary state): Anxiety for others

For those who suffer uncertainty:
- *Cerato* (core remedy): Needs others for advice and confirmation
- *Scleranthus* (core remedy): Indecision
- *Gentian* (core remedy): Doubt and discouragement
- *Gorse* (helper remedy): Hopelessness

- *Hornbeam* (temporary state): Mental fatigue
- *Wild Oat* (helper remedy): Lack of motivation and incentive

Not sufficient interest in present circumstances:

- *Clematis* (core remedy): Indifference or boredom
- *Honeysuckle* (temporary state): Living in the past
- *Wild Rose* (temporary state): Feeling of powerlessness
- *Olive* (helper remedy): Mental/emotional and physical weakness
- *White Chestnut* (temporary state): Lack of mental tranquility

Loneliness:

- *Water Violet* (core remedy): Pride or aloofness
- *Impatience* (core remedy): Impatience
- *Heather* (helper remedy): Self-centered, loquacious

Oversensitive to influences and ideas:

- *Agrimony* (core remedy): Mental torture or worry
- *Centaury* (core remedy): Weak willed, subservient
- *Walnut* (temporary state): Easily impressionable, old habits die-hard
- *Holly* (helper remedy): Hatred, envy, and jealousy

Despondency and Despair:

- *Larch* (temporary state): Low self-esteem
- *Pine* (temporary state): Guilt and self-blame
- *Elm* (temporary state): Feeling overwhelmed
- *Sweet Chestnut* (temporary state): Extreme anguish
- *Star of Bethlehem* (temporary state): Sadness, grief, and shock
- *Willow* (temporary state): Resentment and bitterness
- *Oak* (helper remedy): Despondency from overwork
- *Crab Apple* (temporary state): Shame, sense of uncleanliness

Over care for welfare of others:

- *Chicory* (core remedy): Over concern for welfare of others
- *Vervain* (core remedy): Tenseness, over anxiety, over enthusiasm
- *Vine* (helper remedy): Domination over others
- *Beech* (temporary state): Intolerance, over critical
- *Rock Water* (helper remedy): Self-repression and denial

Four Basic ways of using the Flower Remedies

- *Prevention:* use as mental/emotional states arise
- *Stop illness at onset:* treat mental/emotional component accompanying onset of illness
- *Help during illness once illness starts:* used to lift emotions, ease the pain and discomfort
- *Help correct character traits that bring unhappiness:* used to transform undesirable traits into positive aspects that allow for increased personal growth and interpersonal relations

The beautiful feature of using Bach's flower essences is that they work subtly without stressing the patient. The energy pattern of each flower essence causes a change in the vibrational frequencies of the brain's thought processes. The patient then is forced to deal with the situation he or she has been unable to resolve. The big advantage is that there are zero side effects with this type of therapy. Required dosage is usually two to four drops of liquid taken three or four times a day either under the tongue or mixed in bottled water. Again selection of the appropriate remedy can be done through a questionnaire or more accurately autonomic response testing can be used. Within the last year I have been using cranial rhythm as a means of selecting the correct remedy. In my clinical experience, this later technique is the most accurate since the practitioner is using the body's own computer to make the selection.

Bach Flower Essences are available from ICNR, Inc. 1-800-272-2323 or ordered on-line at: *www.icnr.com*

PHARMACEUTICAL PREPARATIONS

The use of pharmaceutical drugs to treat anxiety and depression in cancer patients posses a major potential hazard. Most if not all cancer patients are toxic (build-up of chemical poisons: fluoride, chlorine, PCBs, pesticides, artificial food colorings, prolonged use of prescription drugs and drug metabolites; heavy metals from mercury dental fillings, infections from root canalled teeth, tonsils or jaw bone infections and constipation) even before the cancer develops. This toxic state contributed to the ultimate breakdown of the immune system in the first place. The cancer patient's liver and kidneys are already over burdened removing toxic wastes produced by the cancer cells, plus the daily intake burden of chemicals, over-processed foods, additives, colorings and "synthetic vitamin enriched" foods. What the body needs less of is additional chemical poisons and intermediary metabolites from drugs. Just read the PDR – Physicians Desk Reference on all the warnings and potential side effects of these medications.

Diazepam (Valium) Valium belongs to the family of drugs Benzodiazepines. These drugs are generally classified as minor tranquilizers useful for short-term management of anxiety. It may also be used to treat symptoms of acute alcohol withdrawals, to help control epilepsy, or to relieve muscle spasms. Benzodiazepines include drugs such as Librium® (chlordiazepoxide), Serax® (oxazepam), Ativan® (lorazepam), Xanax® (alprazolam), and Clonopin® (clonazepam).

Description: In addition to the active ingredient diazepam, each tablet contains the following inactive ingredients: anhydrous lactose, corn starch, pre-gelatinized starch and calcium stearate with the following dyes: 5-mg tablets contain FD&C Yellow No. 6 and D&C Yellow No. 10; 10-mg tablets contain FD&C Blue No. 1. Valium 2-mg tablets contain no dye.

Warnings Narcotics may increase the sedative effects of this drug. Do not take other sedatives, benzodiazepines, or sleeping pills with this drug. The combinations could be fatal. Do not drink alcohol when taking benzodiazepines. Alcohol can lower blood pressure and decrease your breathing rate to the point of unconsciousness.

- The habit-forming potential is high. It is possible to become dependent in only two weeks. These drugs should not be taken for more then four weeks (Yudofsky, Hales and Ferguson). Do not stop taking this drug abruptly; this could cause psychological and physical withdrawal symptoms.

- Do not take this drug if you are pregnant. Some studies have found that taking this drug may lead to serious birth defects. If this drug is used in late pregnancy it may cause "floppy infant" syndrome.

- Do not take this drug if planning to become pregnant. Do not take if you are breast-feeding.

- Do not give this drug to anyone under six months old and never use on hyperactive or psychotic children. Only use drug in small doses if over sixty with close monitoring.

Do not use if: You had negative reactions to other benzodiazepines, if you have a history of drug dependence, if you have had a stroke, if you have multiple sclerosis, if you have Alzheimer's disease, if you are seriously depressed or if you have other brain disorders.

In elderly and debilitated patients, it is recommended that the dosage be limited to the smallest effective amount to preclude the development of ataxia (inability to co-ordinate voluntary bodily movements) or over-sedation (2 mg to 2.5 mg once or twice daily, initially, to be increased gradually as needed and tolerated).

Common Side Effects: Clumsiness or unsteadiness; dizziness or lightheadedness; drowsiness; slurred speech.

Less Common or Rare Side Effects: Abdominal or stomach cramps or pain; blurred vision or other changes in vision; changes in sexual desire or ability; constipation; diarrhea; dry mouth or increased thirst; false sense of well-being; headache; increased bronchial secretions or watering of mouth; muscle spasm; nausea or vomiting; problems with urination; trembling or shaking; unusual tiredness or weakness.

Always Notify Doctor:

Less Common: Anxiety; confusion (may be more common in the elderly); fast, pounding, or irregular heartbeat; lack of memory of events after benzodiazepine is taken (may be more common with triazolam); depression.

Rare: Abnormal thinking, including disorientation, delusions (holding false beliefs that cannot be changed by facts), or loss of sense of reality; agitation; behavior changes, including aggressive behavior, bizarre behavior, decreased inhibition, or outbursts of anger; convulsions (seizures); hallucinations (seeing, hearing, or feeling things that are not there); hypotension (low blood pressure); muscle weakness; skin rash or itching; sore throat, fever and chills; trouble sleeping; ulcers or sores in mouth or throat (continuing); uncontrolled movements of body, including the eyes; unusual bleeding or bruising; unusual excitement, nervousness, or irritability; unusual tiredness or weakness (severe); yellow eyes or skin.

Stop taking and see physician Immediately: Convulsions, hallucinations, memory loss, trouble breathing or staggering/trembling.

SSRIs (SELECTIVE SEROTONIN UPTAKE INHIBITORS)

The next generation of anti-depressant drugs started appearing in 1988 with the introduction of Prozac. The strategy behind these SSRI drugs was to develop a medication with pharmacologic "intelligence", that is, a substance capable of affecting specific sites of action (uptake receptor areas) while avoiding effects on other sites, which are responsible for causing adverse side effects. The goal of these so-called "smart" drugs was to produce agents that were more efficacious, safer and better tolerated than the older medications. In theory, this intelligent evolution of designer drugs appeared promising. Additional medications within this SSRI group started appearing in the 1990's. Prozac, Paxil, Zoloft, Celexa and Lexapro.

The following overview on the SSRI drugs is to alert the patient and or caregiver of information that may have been omitted by the treating physician. Portions of the information supplied have been excerpted from a continuing education lecture for physicians presented by James L. Schaller, MD. His web site *www.personalconsult.com* provides timely information for anyone seeking altenative solutions to psychiatric and anti-aging problems.

After reviewing 11 million references in Pubmed and 127 published reports of SSRI-induced movement disorders of Zoloft, Paxil and Prozac, Dr. Schaller concluded, "*All major anti-depressants have muscle disorders and movement disorders, except citalopram (Celexa) or escitalopram (Lexapro).*" Schaller also noted that Canadian manufacturers reported almost one thousand cases. Canada's pharmaceutical manufacture's list of unpublished reports on SSRI-induced side effects:

- *Akathisia* – 49 cases – excessive, usually repetitive, movements such as pacing, foot tapping and rocking. Also refers to a subjective inner agitation.
- *Dystonia* – 44 cases – muscle spasms.

- *Dyskinesia* – 208 cases – faulty perception of sensation of motion or position.
- *Tardive Dyskinesia* – 76 cases – involuntary movement and twitching of the face muscles.
- *Parkinsonism* – 516 cases – tremors, rigid muscles, difficulty moving and unresponsive expression.
- *Bruxism* – 60 cases – repetitive grinding of the teeth.
(Annals of Pharmacotherapy 1998;32:692)

The significance of the issue of various anti-depressant SSRI-induced movement disorders is not of secondary importance. Doctor Schaller's impression is that SSRI-induced akathisia is incorrectly perceived, and diagnosed as:

- Anxiety disorders
- Onset side effects of the medication
- New stressors
- Panic disorder
- Anxiety from Major Depression
- Anesthesia effects

If a person is slowed down from Parkinson's Disease the akathisia will not be observable. (Akathasia masked by hypokinesia. Pharmacopsychiatry 2000;33:147-9)

Anti-Depressants have different movement disorder frequencies. One example: Remission of SSRI-induced akathisia after switching to another anti-depressant medication, nefazodone (Serzone). (J of Clinical Psychiatry 2001;62:570). The irony of this drug shell game is that another medication was used to eliminate one drug-induced side effect, akathisia, with another drug, Serzone, which the FDA recognizes as being linked to causing liver failure!

Anti-depressant Serzone Linked To Life-Threatening Liver Failure, Zimmerman, Reed, PLLP:" On December 7, 2001, the Food and Drug Administration informed Bristol-Meyers Squib Co. that it must include a "black-box" warning on the labels of a popular anti-depressant called *SERZONE.* This warning came after it was learned that *SERZONE* was responsible for life-threatening liver failures that led to death or the necessity of a liver transplant. *A black-box designation is reserved for only the most serious side effects in medications.* SERZONE had been considered an important alternative to the top-selling class of anti-depressants, because it is often regarded as less disruptive to sexual activity than Zoloft, Paxil or Prozac."

Serzone has now been recalled in Europe and Now Canada! Serzone has been taken off the market because it has been linked to many deaths resulting from liver damage. *According to the manufacturer, the rate of liver failure in SERZONE users is about 3 to 4 times greater than in non-users.*

The Complexities of Akathisia:

- Akathisia increases depression
- Akathisia hinders attention
- Akathisia causes cognitive problems

(Subjective emotional experience and cognitive impairment in drug-induced akathisia. Comprehensive Psychiatry 2002;43:456-62 & the symptomology of akathisia. Fortschr Neurol Psychiatr 1997;65:232-6)

To underscore the significance of the SSRI-induced side effects and the risks of taking these designer drugs, the following case study and literature citation are presented: The *Journal of Clinical Psychiatry* (1996:57:449) discusses 71 cases of SSRI-induced neurologic symptoms (extrapyramidal stimulation) of which 75% were attributed to the use of Prozac (fluoxetine). The 71 cases reviewed provided the following symptom groups:

- Akathisia 45%
- Dystonia 28%
- Parkinsonism 14%
- Tardive Dyskinesia-like state 11%

Case 1: 72-year-old woman with rhythmic palatal movements, chorea (brief, irregular contractions that are not repetitive or rhythmic, but appear to flow from one muscle to the next) and possibly muscle spasm while on Prozac (fluoxetine) which stopped after 5 days when the drug was discontinued.

Case 2: 56-year-old male with rapid patterned toe movements while on Prozac and resolved with discontinued use. (Movement Disorders 1996;11:324). Acute muscle spasm caused by Prozac (Medical Clinics Barc 1992:99:436)

Warning: When selective serotonin reuptake inhibitors are taken with non-steroidal anti-inflammatory drugs (NSAIDs: Daypro, Feldene, Nuprin, Naprosyn, Motrin (Ibuprofen), Vioxx), Tylenol or aspirin, the risk of bleeding is greatly increased. They say that this finding may have important public health implications owing to the high prevalence of both anti-depressants and NSAIDs in most developed countries.

Greater caution is probably warranted in co-administering non-steroidal anti-inflammatory drugs (NSAIDs) and serotonin reuptake inhibitors."

Prozac (fluoxetine) Prozac is used to treat depression, obsessive compulsive disorder (OCD), and eating disorders.

Prozac's link to suicidal tendencies: In the early 1990's, Eli Lilly, the manufacturer of Prozac, discerned such a pattern in the reported Prozac suicides and identified four distinctive attributes of this puzzling paradox:

- the patients became *SUDDENLY SUICIDAL,* usually within the first 30 days of taking the drug or increasing their dose;
- the suicide attempts were all *VIOLENT,* even those by women;
- the patient's actions before and during the suicidal act were *OBSESSIVE* or impulsive in nature; and
- the suicide was completely *OUT OF CHARACTER,* or "egodystonic."

Liver Disease: Because of its crucial role in metabolism, liver impairment can affect the elimination of fluoxetine. In patients with alcohol-induced cirrhosis, the elimination half-life of fluoxetine was prolonged, with a mean of 7.6 days compared to 2 to 3 days seen in subjects without liver disease. Norfluoxetine elimination half-life was also delayed, with a mean duration of 12 days for cirrhotic patients compared to 7 to 9 days in normal subjects. *This suggests that the use of fluoxetine in patients with liver disease must be approached with caution.* Why hasn't any research been done on the withholding of Prozac in cancer patients?

Prozac's primary indication is for the *symptomatic* relief of depressive illness. Most physicians who prescribe Prozac are not aware of the fact that Fluoxetine has three molecules of fluoride in its chemical structure (Prozac (Fluoxetine Hydrochloride) is designated:(+-)-N-methyl-3-phenyl-3-((a,a,a)-*trifluoro-p*-tolyl)oxy) propylamine). Fluoride suppresses the function of the thyroid gland, which can result in depression and anxiety. Physicians should not prescribe a drug that *potentially* causes the same problem the medication is trying to alleviate. Conventional medicine focuses on symptomatic relief! To truly heal, the underlying cause must be uncovered and corrected.

Implications of the Long Elimination Half-Life of Fluoxetine: Because of the long elimination half-lives of fluoxetine and its major active metabolite norfluoxetine, changes in dose will not be fully reflected in plasma for several weeks, affecting both strategies for maintaining a final dose and withdrawal from treatment. Even when dosing is stopped, the *active drug substance will persist in the body for five weeks due to the long elimination half-lives of fluoxetine and norfluoxetine.* This is of potential consequence when drug discontinuation is required or when drugs are prescribed that might interact with fluoxetine and norfluoxetine following discontinuation of fluoxetine.

It is obvious that this drug has the potential to further damage an already compromised liver. And most cancer patients are not in the best of health. The last thing they need is more poison in their system and more symptoms to deal with.

Check with your doctor if any of the following side effects continue or are bothersome:

- *Most Common Side Effects of Prozac:* Anxiety or nervousness; decreased appetite; diarrhea; drowsiness; headache; increased sweating; nausea; tiredness or weakness; trembling or shaking; trouble sleeping.

- *Less Common or Rare Side Effects of Prozac:* Abnormal dreams; change in sense of taste; changes in vision; chest pain; constipation; dizziness or lightheadedness; dryness of mouth; feeling of warmth or heat; flushing or redness of skin, especially on face and neck; frequent urination; hair loss; increased appetite; increased sensitivity of skin to sunlight; menstrual pain; stomach cramps, gas, or pain; vomiting; weight loss; yawning.

- *Rare Side Effects:* Rare: Breast enlargement or pain; convulsions (seizures); fast or irregular heartbeat; purple or red spots on skin; symptoms of hypoglycemia (low blood sugar), including anxiety or nervousness, chills, cold sweats, confusion, cool pale skin, difficulty in concentration, drowsiness, excessive hunger, fast heartbeat, headache, shakiness or unsteady walk, unusual tiredness or weakness; symptoms of hyponatremia (low blood sodium), including confusion, convulsions (seizures), drowsiness, dry mouth, increased thirst, lack of energy; symptoms of serotonin syndrome, include diarrhea, fever, increased sweating, mood or behavior changes, overactive reflexes, racing heartbeat, restlessness, shivering or shaking; talking, feeling, and acting with uncontrollable excitement and activity; trouble breathing; unusual or incomplete body or facial movements; unusual secretion of milk in females.

- Fluoxetine and extrapyramidal side effects (American J. Psychiatry 1996;153:449).

- Fluoxetine and extrapyramidal side effects (American J. Psychiatry 1989;146:1352).

- Persistent dyskinesia in a patient receiving fluoxetine (American J Psychiatry 1991;148:1403).

- Fluoxetine induced dyskinesia case with rapid onset and cessation after stopping fluoxetine (Aust N Z J Psychiatry 1994;28:328).

- Fluoxetine associated dystonia (American J Psychiatry 1994;151:149).

- Acute dystonia and fluoxetine (J. Clinical Psychiatry 1992;53:327).

- Fluoxetine-related indifference and akathisia. A case report (Therapie 1993;48:158).

Paxil (Paroxetine HCl) In just a few years, Paxil has become one of the leading treatments for depression and anxiety disorders in the country. This medication is used to treat depression, panic attacks, obsessive compulsive disorders (OCD), social anxiety disorder (social phobia), and generalized anxiety disorder. Paxil works by helping to restore the balance of certain natural chemicals in the brain. Paxil CR is a controlled (timed) release form of Paxil.

Side Effects of Paxil:

- A common side effect of Paxil is nausea, which may be lessened by taking it with food.

- Other side effects may include injury, infection, diarrhea, constipation, decreased appetite, sleepiness, dizziness, yawning, sweating, abnormal vision, and sexual side effects.

- Meaningful weight gain.

- Paxil and Prozac have higher incidence of drug interactions than other SSRI drugs.
- Increased incidence of breast cancer: usually occurs two years after discontinued use.; based on personal communication with Dr. James L. Schaller
- If you should *experience any side effects, be sure to report them to your healthcare provider as soon as possible and follow his/her advice.*

On June 19, 2003, the FDA warned that the popular anti-depressant "Paxil", which is manufactured by British pharmaceutical giant GlaxoSmithKline, should not be given to depressed children 18 and under because of an increased *RISK OF SUICIDE.*

England has recently banned the use of Paxil for children and teenagers under the age of 18 because the drug has been linked to suicide, suicidal behavior and violent outbursts.

GlaxoSmithKline has updated its labeling text to include akathisia as a primary drug-induced side effect. Although there are several biologically plausible precursors of SSRI-induced violence/suicide, akathisia is the neurological condition, which has been most implicated in the numerous scientific articles linking all of the SSRI drugs to these violent acts.

"Serotonin-specific reuptake inhibitor antidepressant medications may produce akathisia" … "the subjective distress resulting from akathisia … may be associated with … irritability, aggression, or suicide attempts."

Prior to these revisions numerous world class experts, including Teicher & Cole, Mann & Kapur, Wirshing & Van Putten, and Dr. David Healy and his colleagues in the UK, had warned about the role of SSRI-induced akathisia in violence and suicide since the early 1990's. Moreover, an extensive 1997 review article by Pfizer's own Dr. Roger Lane confirmed that this precursor to violence/suicide is caused by *all* of the *SSRI drugs,* including his company's Zoloft. In spite of this wealth of information, however, the big drug companies continued to *deny the causal relationship and to conceal evidence of same in unpublished data and in documents hidden from public scrutiny by means of "confidentiality" designations in civil litigation.*

The FDA's action came shortly after the two-year anniversary of a federal jury verdict in the *Tobin v. SmithKline Beecham* case. After considering extensive evidence from both sides, the jury found that "Paxil can cause *some people* to become homicidal and/or suicidal" and that it caused a peaceful, family man named Donald Schell to shoot his wife, daughter, granddaughter, and then himself. The judge ruled that the verdict was supported by scientifically reliable, legally admissible evidence and entered a $6.4 million judgment for the clients.

GlaxoSmithKline's new "Dear Doctor" letter implicitly confirms, *Paxil can trigger violent and suicidal actions in both children and adults. The numerous articles on point include Dr. J. John Mann's 1991 article alerting the profession to the possibilities of iatragenic suicide in a "small vulnerable subpopulation" of patients.*

Mann and Kapur, *The Emergence of Suicidal Ideation and Behavior During Antidepressant Pharmacotherapy,* 48 Arch. Gen. Psych. 1027-33 (1991). Dr. Mann has served as a consultant for Eli Lilly and as a paid litigation expert witness for both Pfizer and SmithKline Beecham.

As a paid expert witness for both Pfizer and SmithKline Beecham, Dr. Mann has confirmed that akathisia does increase the risk of suicidality.

Finally, there is little question about the fact that the dangers of violence and suicide are *common to the entire class of SSRI drugs*. This point is especially critical in view of the fact that both Prozac and Zoloft are being heavily prescribed to children in this country.

Numerous sources document the class-wide nature of these problems. Donovan and colleagues published an epidemiological study in the year 2000. Both Lilly and SmithKline Beecham provided funding for the study. The study evaluated 2776 patients and calculated the risk of "deliberate self-harm" from the SSRI drugs as a class to be 5.5 times higher than the safest of the older, tried and true, tricyclic anti-depressants. Prozac (fluoxetine), Zoloft (sertraline) and Paxil/Seroxat (paroxetine) increase this risk significantly. Interestingly, within the class of SSRI drugs, Prozac had the highest risk at 6.6x and Zoloft the second highest at 4.9x. The risk from Paxil was 4.0 times normal.

References
- Paroxetine and akathisia (Biological Psychiatry 1995;37:336)
- A case of paroxetine-induced akathisia (Biological Psychiatry 1996:39:910)
- Three cases of akathisia were found in 67 patients treated with paroxetine at Mass. General. (Akathisia: a review and case report following paroxetine treatment. Comprehensive Psychiatry 1996:37:122-4). 1/22 patients.
- Paroxetine and tardive akathisia (Canadian J Psychiatry 2000;45:398)
- Paroxetine and tardive dyskinesia (J Clinical Psychopharmacology 1996;16:258-9)
- A case of paroxetine-induced dyskinetic movements (J Clinical Psychopharmacol 2000;20:712-3)
- Parkinsonism exacerbated by paroxetine. (Neurology 1994;44:2406)
- Tourette's syndrome and antidepressant therapy: exacerbation of nervous tics with paroxetine (Z Kinder Jugendpsychiatr Psychther 2000;28:105-8)

Zoloft (Sertraline) Zoloft is used to treat depression, panic attacks, obsessive compulsive disorders (OCD), and post-traumatic stress disorder (PTSD). Zoloft works by helping to restore the balance of certain natural chemicals in the brain. Zoloft has also been used to treat a severe form of premenstrual syndrome (premenstrual dysphoric disorder – PMDD) and a sexual function problem in men (premature ejaculation).

Side effects associated with Zoloft: Dry mouth, feeling or being sick, loss of appetite, upset stomach, diarrhea, abdominal pain, shaky feeling (tremor), sweating, change in sex drive or function e.g. ejaculatory delay, dizziness, not being able to sleep, excessive sleepiness, indigestion. All medicines can cause allergic reactions. Serious allergic reactions are rare. Any sudden wheezing, difficulty breathing, swelling, rash or itching (especially affecting the whole body), a vague feeling of being unwell, tiredness, joint or muscle pain.

Effects associated with depression: anxiety, unable to sleep, crying, tingling or numbness, convulsions, confusion, amnesia, uncontrollable twitching, jerking or writhing movements (more likely if you already experience such effects) mania/ hypomania, hallucinations, abnormalities in liver function tests.

Rarely: jaundice, inflammation of the pancreas or liver, liver failure, lower sodium content of the blood; increase in the hormone prolactin, which could lead to symptoms such as abnormal production of breast milk or breast enlargement, menstrual irregularities, skin rash and sensitivity to sunlight, agitation, aggression; symptoms such as dizziness, tingling, headache, anxiety and nausea may occur if Zoloft treatment is stopped too quickly.

Warning: Do not take Zoloft within 2 weeks of taking any drug classified as an MAO inhibitor. Drugs in this category include the antidepressants Marplan, Nardil, and Parnate. When serotonin boosters such as Zoloft are combined with MAO inhibitors, serious and sometimes fatal reactions can occur.

Based on the clinical data compiled by James L. Schaller, MD, MAR, PA, DABPN, DABFM, blood levels of Zoloft go down every year even though a maximum daily dose of 200mg is maintained.

Several published analyses of FDA data by other independent analysts have clearly demonstrated that there exists no credible evidence from controlled clinical trials that these drugs are any more effective than placebo-only that they produce an effect. For that reason, the risks posed by these drugs must be fully justified. Contrary to denials by the drug makers, psychiatrists who are paid by these companies, and until now, denial by FDA officials, there IS credible evidence that Paxil, Prozac, Zoloft and the other SSRIs cause suicide and/or aggression. As the powerful investigative reports by the BBC revealed that there is also credible evidence of severe withdrawal symptoms- a sign of addiction.

Possible food and drug interactions when taking this medication: You should not drink alcoholic beverages while taking Zoloft. Use over-the-counter remedies with caution. Although none is known to interact with Zoloft, interactions remain a possibility.

If Zoloft is taken with certain other drugs, the effects of one or the other could be increased, decreased, or altered. It is especially important to check with your doctor before combining Zoloft with the following:

- Cimetidine (Tagamet)
- Diazepam (Valium)
- Digitoxin (Crystodigin)
- Flecainide (Tambocor)
- Lithium (Eskalith, Lithobid)

- MAO inhibitor drugs such as the antidepressants Nardil and Parnate
- Other serotonin-boosting drugs such as Paxil and Prozac
- Other antidepressants such as Elavil and Serzone
- Over-the-counter drugs such as cold remedies
- Propafenone (Rythmol)
- Sumatriptan (Imitrex)
- Tolbutamide (Orinase)
- Warfarin (Coumadin)
- If you are using the oral concentrate form of Zoloft, do not take disulfiram (Antabuse)

Celexa and Lexapro Celexa was introduced in 1988. It is an antidepressant that is also a member of the family of drugs known as selective serotonin reuptake inhibitors (SSRIs). Celexa helps to restore the brain's chemical balance by increasing the supply of a substance in the brain called serotonin. Celexa appears to relieve depression by increasing serotonin without affecting many of the other chemicals in the brain that influence mood. Celexa has been made into a purified form, Lexapro, which has fewer side effects. *Lexapro's Superiority is Worth a Very Serious Look For Treatment of Major Depression.*

Caution: Starting dose of 5 mg is too high. At this dose nausea and headaches frequently occur. A dose of 2.5 mg is recommended.

One of the big advantages of using Lexapro is that it presents the least burden to the liver.

- Drug interaction's kill during suicides and routine medication use. Lexapro has the lowest interactions of all SSRIs including Zoloft. Interaction materials are merely fair. None are fully reliable. Yet jury's think interactions are always the physician's fault, and if they occur are due to carelessness and "not caring."
- All SSRIs cause akathisia, extrapyramidal stimulation, Tardive Dyskinesia, and Dystonia. Celexa and Lexapro have no reports of these problems. Disparity of cases is not due to difference in articles, e.g., Celexa/Lexapro have more publications than Sertraline (Zoloft).
- Anxiety is a massive independent risk factor for suicide. Depression already has a suicide rate of 15/100. Lexapro and Celexa have the lowest onset anxiety rate, the lowest akathisia rate and the fastest anxiety reduction.
- Paxil and Prozac have *Non-Linear* Kinetics, so you also have "surprise" *Non-Linear Interactions.*
- All hormones, drugs and toxins require internal liver detox substances to remove them. EPA 1986 Adipose tissue study showed all of us have at least 5 major toxins in our fat. Obviously average people are failing at removing dangerous substances. One liver detox agent, glutathione, is used up by mere Tylenol. *Chemotherapy empties the liver of detox agents.*

- Lexapro is a *pure select isomer and only usable medication* — less of a liver load. Allowing the liver to remove more serious substances.
- Weight gain with Lexapro vs. Other SSRIs:
  a. Paxil has meaningful weight gain. 25.5% of patients taking Paxil for a period ranging from 26-32 weeks exhibited a weight gain greater than 7%. (Fava M, et al. J Clin Psychiatry. 2000;61:863-867)
  b. Other medications which increase norepinephine appear to increase glucose levels and increase insulin resistance.
  c. Anxiety onset symptoms or under-treated anxiety increases eating as a coping mechanism.
- Increased anxiety is a key feature of PMS/PDD and Perimenopause. All are characterized, in part, by decreased natural progesterone. Decreased progesterone increases anxiety (GABA) and increases pain (via 2 pain networks). Therefore, if one is committed to an SSRI for these problems it should be Lexapro; lowest onset anxiety, fast decrease in anxiety and no known akathisia.
- Lexapro does not interact with over a 100 important receptors.
- You should not take Celexa if you are currently taking certain other antidepressant medications in the group called monoamine oxidase (MAO) inhibitors, such as phenelzine or tranylcypromine. You should stop taking MAO inhibitors 2 weeks before starting Celexa, and you should be off Celexa for 2 weeks before starting on MAO inhibitor medication.

General Precautions with Celexa:
- Do not drive or operate heavy machinery until you know how you will react to Celexa.
- Drinking alcohol while being treated with Celexa is not recommended.

If you currently have, or have a history of the following conditions, your health care provider will evaluate you to decide if Celexa is right for you:
- Mania
- Seizures
- Liver disease
- Severe kidney problems

The most common side effect with Celexa is sexual problems in male patients.

Some other possible side effects include:
- Nausea
- Dry mouth
- Sleepiness
- Increase in sweating

The following table provides a quick overview of Drug-Drug Interactions:

DRUG-DRUG INTERACTIONS			
Celexa	Mild	Minimal	Minimal	Minimal
Lexapro	Minimal	Minimal	Minimal	Minimal
Prozac	Mild	Mild/Moderate	Strong	Moderate
Paxil	Mild	Mild	Strong	Minimal
Zoloft	Mild	Mild/Moderate	Minimal	Minimal

EXAMPLES OF DRUGS AFFECTED			
Theophylline	Phenytoin	Tramadol	Carbamazepine
Warfarin	Warfarin	Codeine	Corticosteroids
Amitriptyline	Zolpidem	Corticosteroids	Olanzapine
Acetaminophen (Tylenol)	Omeprazole	Trazodone	Cyclosporine
Caffeine	Captopril	Resperidone	Nifedipine
	Celecoxib	Haloperidol	Alprazolam
	Propranolol	Digitoxin	

Greenblatt DJ. J Clin Psychopharm.1999;19 (suppl 1):23S-35S

Hesse L. Drug Metab Dispos. 2000;28:1176-1183

Stomer E. Drug Metab Dispos. 2000;28:1168-1175

Michalets EL. Pharmacotherapy. 1998;18:84-112

Cupp MJ. Amer Fam Physician. 1998;57:107-116

Pichard L. Drug Metab Dispos. 1995;23:1253-1262

von Moltke LL, et al. Drug Metab Dispos. 2001;29:1102-1108

Information taken from Larry Culpepper, MD, MPH lecture notes.

How good is America's drug safety system? Since 1997, more than a dozen prescription drugs have been taken off the market due to serious side effects — in some cases after hundreds of injuries and even deaths have occurred. Is the Food and Drug Administration, which is responsible for approving and monitoring the safety of the medications we take, up to the task? Sidney Wolfe, MD, director of Public Citizen's Health Research Group, in response to the FDA's present state of affairs, made the following statement.

"In the 31 years that I've been monitoring the Food and Drug Administration, what has gone on in the last five and six years is unprecedented. There have been an unprecedented number and percentage of drugs taken off the market; in many cases, drugs with known problems before they came on the market.

"There's an unprecedented turnover of top scientists and physicians at the FDA. We now have three former FDA scientists on our staff. The absence of congressional oversight to sort of hold the FDA accountable has also been devastating. So the outcome of all of this is that we've had more drug safety-related problems in the last four or five years than really almost any comparable period of time.

"The sad thing is these were preventable. They could have been avoided. In most, if not all of the cases, there were strong danger signals even before the drug came on the market that there was a problem. In all cases, once they came on the market, there was a very dangerous and reckless slowness to respond to the signals that came after marketing — signals in the terms of deaths and serious injuries to people who took the drug once it was on the market. So I think the combination of problems in the pre-approval phase, combined with a very defective system for post-market safety surveillance have really been devastating.

"At one time, 10 years ago, I would have said — and did say — that the FDA was the gold standard, that no country was doing a better job, either in the approval of drugs in the first place, or, secondly, in finding out as quickly as possible once they came on the market. That's no longer the case. Other countries that formerly were looking up to our gold standard are now outperforming us, and protecting people in those countries much more than we are protecting Americans. ..."

If SSRIs or other antidepressant medications are not alleviating the anxiety or depression, patients and/or caregivers must contact the treating physician. Further evaluation will be needed to select alternative medicines and with fewer potential side effects or explore alternative substances. Weaning oneself off SSRIs to prevent *Discontinuation Syndrome* is a topic most physicians are ill equipped to handle. The following information is provided by Paula Host and is one of the best approaches available.

"You've been on an SSRI antidepressant for five weeks or more. The doctor feels that the dosage needs to be decreased or the medication needs to be discontinued. He prescribes changes and tapering in the usual 10mg increments.

"Within a couple of days of starting this, you begin to exhibit severe flu like symptoms — headache, diarrhea, nausea, vomiting, chills, dizziness and fatigue. There may be insomnia. Agitation, impaired concentration, vivid dreams, depersonalization, irritability and suicidal thoughts are sometimes occurring. "These symptoms last anywhere from one to seven weeks and vary in intensity. You wonder what the heck is going on.

"It's called SSRI discontinuation syndrome, and it can really be the pits. Here is what causes it:

"Some SSRI medications have a very short half-life. This means they produce no metabolites that help the medication stay in the body for an extended period. They go in, last a few hours, and come out again.

"SSRIs are split into two categories: long acting and short acting. For example, Prozac is a longer-acting SSRI. Paxil, Effexor, Zoloft and Luvox are short-acting. The shorter acting SSRIs, when discontinued or when the dosage is lowered, produce an "anti-cholinergic rebound," which is an interruption in production of the key neurotransmitter acetylcholine. (Acetylcholine is the neurotransmitter used more when a person is under greater stress.) These symptoms will last anywhere from one to seven weeks, and then disappear.

Neurologic symptoms include:

- Dizziness
- Vertigo
- Lightheadedness
- Difficulty walking

Somatic (bodily) complaints include:

- Nausea/vomiting
- Fatigue
- Headaches
- Insomnia

Less common difficulties:

- Shock-like sensations
- Parasthesia (skin crawling, burning or prickling)
- Visual disturbances
- Diarrhea
- Muscle pain
- Chills

Non-specific mental symptoms:

- Shock-like sensations
- Agitation
- Impaired concentration
- Vivid dreams
- Depersonalization — sense of unreality and loss of self
- Irritability
- Suicidal thoughts

"Double-blind controlled studies now indicate that 35-78% of patients, who, after five weeks or more of treatment with the medication, abruptly stop certain antidepressants or titrate down in 10mg increments or more, will develop one or more of the discontinuation symptoms. When allowed to run its course, the syndrome duration is variable (one to several weeks) and ranges from mild-moderate intensity in most patients, to extremely distressing in a small number.

Practical Tips for Tapering Off

(Wisdom from Paula HOST)

- "So ... you are using a short-acting SSRI medication. You have to discontinue it or titrate it down, you tend to be very sensitive to the effects of medication withdrawal, and you want to know what to do to head off discontinuation syndrome?

- "First, ask your doctor if a special dose is available for the specific purpose of weaning down. Some pharmaceutical companies are now manufacturing and offering them in sample form to doctors. Ask.

- "If such a dose is not available, the main thing to remember is that you want to try and wean down very slowly — usually in half the increments that your doctor would normally suggest for the weaning process in most people.

- "If you have tablets, and the insert doesn't indicate that splitting or crushing is taboo, you can split them (a pill splitter helps, a couple of bucks at the pharmacy). *ALWAYS* check the insert or a drug monograph first to make sure you can split them. This makes it pretty easy to halve the original titration recommendation and take each step down for a week.

"If you have capsules, you have a different type of problem ... you obviously can't open them and take the contents raw...but you can still taper off. Buy some empty gel caps (very cheap — a couple bucks for a hundred). Take a single 24-hour dosage and set it aside. Open your capsules and redistribute the medication into the empty gel caps to spread the total 24-hour dosage into smaller increments. Rub each capsule prior to storing with a dry cloth to get any of the medication off of the outside of the capsule. There is a little tool that can help you with this if you have pain in your hands or motor problems. You then set a 24-hour dosage amount aside, and gradually reduce it, using each amount for a week.

"I had great success using this method when titrating down from Paxil, one of the most notorious drugs for causing DS. My doctor refused to acknowledge the discontinuation problem and couldn't seem to give me any helpful suggestions for reducing the discomfort. So I did it this way, and the effects were much more tolerable.

"The main thing is that the brain's production of acetylcholine is not interrupted. One of the simplest things you can do to prevent this in addition to ultra-slow titration is to add supplements: in particular, choline, lecithin, and B-complex. The B vitamins will help sustain your brain's current levels of the neurotransmitter acetylcholine (the depletion of which is the cause of DS). You should also use choline supplements or lecithin supplements (which are 13 percent choline) to help increase the level of available choline that the brain uses to make acetylcholine while the titration or discontinuation is happening. (Standard Process provides food-based forms of choline, lecithin and B-complex vitamins. Available from ICNR, Inc. 1-800-272-2323 or order on the web *www.icnr.com*)

"Dietary changes (temporary if you wish until after the med is weaned) can also be made. Lecithin and choline can be found in a wide variety of foods, but many of the richest sources are foods also high in cholesterol and fat. Egg yolks are one of the best dietary sources of lecithin/choline. Other excellent sources of dietary choline are beefsteak, liver, organ meat, spinach, soybeans, cauliflower, wheat germ, peanuts, and brewer's yeast.

"Discontinuation symptoms are not restricted to the SSRIs, as many of you here can attest. Many drugs that act on the central nervous system can cause DS symptoms: monoamine oxidase inhibitors, tricyclic antidepressants, anti-parkinsonian agents, traditional anti-psychotics, and clozapine. Some people have a condition known as rebound, which occurs with the consumption of short acting medications (an agitated state of emotion that occurs at the end of the dosage cycle, and lasts for fifteen or twenty minutes, then disappears). The dietary modifications are helpful for this problem.

"It's good to know that the psychiatric professional community recognizes this phenomenon as valid. Although the symptoms are varied, and are both physical and psychological, a characteristic SSRI discontinuation syndrome is now recognized."

The message is clear and simple. Whenever possible seek out the underlying cause of the problem (hormone imbalances, nutritional deficiencies, neurotransmitter deficiencies, food allergies, intestinal toxicity, etc.) and use alternative substances first since they present the least potential damage to the body.

NUTRITIONAL SUPPORT FOR COPING WITH DISTRESS

Adaptogens Adaptogens are natural plant products that increase the body's ability to cope with internal and external stress factors, and normalize the functions of the organism. They help maintain a stable internal environment known as homeostasis. They are safe and possess few known side effects.

The main effects of adaptogens are an increased availability of energy during the day, a reduction of stress, increased endurance, greater mental alertness, and deep and restful sleep. Also, adaptogens significantly accelerate the recovery process after illness.

In 1936 a researcher, Hans Selye, MD discovered the body's mechanism for dealing with distress. Selye observed that no matter what the stressor, physical, mental or chemical, the body provided the same response.

The three phases of stress progression

- *Alarm phase* – Some new stress factors cause a sudden release of internal stress-hormones – corticosteroids and catecholamines. If the stress is intense it can damage the regulatory systems of the body permanently and immediately (for example, exposure to high levels of nuclear radiation), but if the person takes adaptogens, then it is possible to smoothly progress further to the "adaptation phase".
- *Adaptation phase* – If the stress factor continues (it might be heavy athletic training) the body learns to tolerate the stressful stimulus – "adapt" – and increase its resistance to the stress factor. The "adaptation phase" is usually a safe period. The longer in the "adaptation phase", the better.
- Finally, the *exhaustion phase* appears, when the body fails to fight stress anymore and simply gives up. In this "exhaustion phase", disease symptoms rapidly appear and worsen.

Diseases associated with stress may appear in the first "alarm phase", but they mainly appear in the third "exhaustion phase" when the body cannot fight stress anymore. This third phase usually develops after a period of months or years. Everything depends on the duration of the "adaptation phase." Sometimes the body may be fortunate and escape this third phase altogether, provided it keeps the stress under control. It is possible to do this by taking adaptogens; they can help the patient to stay in the "adaptation phase" for longer periods by increasing the body's stamina. One of the keys to reversing cancer is to remove the underlying factors while the body is in the adaptation phase. As the immune system recovers the body begins to heal itself and the diseased process reverses.

Optygen™ (Rhodiola rosea) Rhodiola rosea has extraordinary pharmacological properties as an anti-mutagen and *anti-depressive agent*. In this respect Rhodiola rosea is much more powerful than other adaptogens. In one study done by O.M. Duhan and colleagues (4), the anti-mutagenic activities of Panax Ginseng and of Rhodiola rosea were compared. It became clear that the extracts of Rhodiola rosea had a higher capacity to counteract gene mutations induced by various mutagens (up to about 90% inhibition in some cases). The *anti-depressive and anti-stress activity* of Golden root (Rhodiola rosea) is higher than that of St. John's Wort, Ginkgo biloba and Panax Ginseng.

One of the greatest things Rhodiola does is enhance mental and physical performance. It has been widely used by Russian athletes and cosmonauts to increase energy. Rhodiola is cardio-protective, normalizing the heart rate immediately after intense exercise. It improves the nervous system and mental functions such as memory, by increasing blood-supply to the muscles and brain, and it also increases protein synthesis[1,2,3]. *Suggested use:* Three to six capsules daily. Available from ICNR, Inc. 1-800-272-2323 or order on line *www.icnr.com*

SELECTED REFERENCES

[1] Maslova L.V. et al. (1994) "The cardioprotective and antiadrenergic activity of an extract of Rhodiola rosea in stress" Eksp Klin Farmakol 57(6): 61-6

[2] Germano, C. et al. (1999) "Arctic root. The powerful new ginseng alternative" Kensington Publ.Corp.

[3] Petkov, V.D. et. al. (1986) "Effects of alcohol aqueous extract from Rhodiola rosea L. roots on learning and memory" Acta Physiol Pharmacol Bulg 12(1): 3-16

[4] Duhan, O.M. et al. (1999) "The antimutagenic activity of biomass extracts from the cultured cells of medicinal plants in the Ames test" Tsitol Genet Nov-Dec 33(6): 19-25

[5] Udintsev SN; et.al. (1991) "The role of humoral factors of regenerating liver in the development of experimental tumours and the effect of Rhodiola rosea extract on this process" Neoplasma;38(3): 323-31

[6] Bocharova OA et.al. (1995) "The effect of a Rhodiola rosea extract on the incidence of recurrences of a superficial bladder cancer (experimental clinical research)" Urol Nefrol (Mosk) Mar-Apr (2): 46-7

[7] Salikhova RA et.al. (1997) "Effect of Rhodiola rosea on the yield of mutation alteration and DNA repair in bone marrow cells". Patol Fiziol Exsp Ter Oct-Dec (4): 22-4

[8] Linh PT et.al. (2000) "Quantitative determination of salidroside and thyrosol from the underground part of Rhodiola rosea by high performance liquid chromatography" Arch Pharm Res Aug 23(4): 349-52 By: John Hyatt, CA

Disclaimer: The ideas, procedures and suggestions contained in this article are intended for informational purposes only. Always consult with your doctor. All materials regarding your health require medical supervision. These statements have not been evaluated by the FDA, and are not intended to diagnose, treat, or cure any disease.

Ashwaganda (Withania) This herb contains naturally occurring steroidal compounds, alkaloids and other phytochemicals that together produce a tonic and adaptogenic effect on the entire body. *Ashwaganda can:*

- encourage healthy response to environmental stresses
- ease the effects of temporary everyday life changes
- promote an overall feeling of well-being
- enhance immune response
- support the body as it ages
- promote normal blood production, and
- promote healthy growth and development in children.

Ingredients: Ashwaganda root 1:2 extract from Withania somnifera root 2.5 g
Suggested Use: Dilute 5 mL (approx. 1 metric teaspoon) in water or juice once per day or as directed.
Source: Medi Herb
Available from: ICNR, Inc. 1-800-272-2323 or order from web site *www.icnr.com*

Contraindications: Not to be used during pregnancy and lactation unless otherwise directed by a qualified health care practitioner.

There are many adaptogenic herbal substances so have a health care practitioner test which one's are compatible. The following is a partial list:

- *Fenugreek:* used in Chinese medicine
- *Panax ginseng:* stimulatory
- *St. Mary's thistle* (Silybum): liver function
- *Dandelion root* (Taraxacum): liver and gall bladder function
- *Hawthorn* (Crataegus): cardiovascular system
- *Ribwort* (Plantago lanceolata): upper respiratory system
- *Mullein* (Verbascum) *and Inula* (Elecampane): chest
- *St. John's Wort* (Hypericum perforatum), *Withania and Turnera* (Damiana): nervous with hormonal symptoms
- *Sweet fennel* (Foeniculum) *and Cardamon* (Cardamonum): digestion
- *Linseed* (Linum), *Psyllium seed* (Plantago psyllium) and *Peppermint* (Mentha): bowel
- *Echinacea, Picrorrhiza* and *Astragalus:* immune system

HERBAL TRANQUILIZERS

HerbVal Supra This formula is a botanical alternative formulation that has been enhanced by concentrated extracts of nature's renowned herbal sedatives — Valerian Root and Kava Kava. Both of these herbs are well-recognized effective relaxants, able to induce strong calmative feelings while improving mental function and sharpening the senses. Their tranquilizing effects are the result of selective neurotropic action on higher brain centers, which suppress and regulate the autonomic nervous system. Only in an encapsulated product such as *HerbVal Supra* could they be so easily combined. This formulation provides mild sedation and tranquilization at the recommended dosage. Although each of the herbs in this blend is a significant relaxant and sedative by itself, they work best in combination. Unlike conventional medicines often prescribed for relaxation purposes, this formulation closely approximates the effect of taking one (1) 20-milligram tablet of Valium™, a commonly prescribed pharmaceutical used for similar purposes. Unlike its pharmaceutical equivalents, however, *HerbVal Supra* contains no benzodiazepines, has no known contraindications or side effects, and is not habit forming.

Purpose of formulation (Botanical nervine and calmative support for problems with anxiety, fear, overwork, hysteria, and other problems aggravated by emotional disturbances.)

Other applications Insomnia, childhood hyperactivity, psychosomatic problems, and general restlessness. Muscle pain, muscle relaxing. PMS pain and cramps.

Form Capsules (600 mg. each)
Herbal ingredients Standardized herbal extracts of valerian root, hops, passionflower, skullcap, black cohosh, and kava kava.
Recommended dosage: Take one (1) or two (2) capsules per day. Herbal action should take place in 20-30 minutes. For best results, at least one (1) capsule should be taken early in the morning on an empty stomach, with a large glass of cold water.

Contraindications: Consult a physician before taking Kava Kava if currently taking anti-anxiety or anti-depressant prescription medication, or if you suffer from Parkinson's disease. Do not mix with alcohol. Consult your physician before using this product if you are pregnant, lactating, have high blood pressure, heart or thyroid disease, diabetes, or are being treated for a serious medical condition. Do not drive when taking this supplement, as drowsiness will result.
Viable Herbal Solutions P.O. Box 969 Morrisville, PA. 19067-0969;
Phone: 1-800-505-9475, 1-215-337-8182, Fax: 1-800-505-9476; 1-215-337-8186;
Email: *vhssales@alternative-medicines.com; www.viableherbalsolutions.com/*

Serenity A soothing blend of herbs, which have a reputed calming effect. Particularly useful when stress or tension is high. This formulation includes Burdock Root, Beth Root, Black Cohosh, Oregon Grape Root and Milkweed.

Source: Hanna Kroeger Herbs

Suggested Use: Two capsules between meals.

Available from: Hanna's Herb Shop 1-800-206-6722

www.kroegerherb.com/

VITAMINS, MINERALS, AMINO ACIDS AND GLANDULARS

Orchex® (Standard Process) This product is half niacinamide, B-6, half aqueous extract of orchic tissue. It has been shown clinically to have an even greater calming effect than niacinamide, B-6, alone. It is one of the strongest nutritional tranquilizers available, used for depression, nervous tension, feelings of insecurity and to help patients calm down when they are in crisis.

Ingredients: Calcium lactate 20 mg, Sodium 25 mg, niacinamide 25mg, pyridoxine B-6 5mg, magnesium citrate, plus each tablet supplies 165 mg bovine orchic PMG™ extract.

Suggested Use: One tablet per meal, or as directed. Contraindications: None

Available from: ICNR, Inc. order from web site *www.icnr.com* or 1-800-272-2323

L-Tryptophan This amino acid is a natural way to increase serotonin production. Serotonin is a mood-elevating neurotransmitter that mediates depression. Other common symptoms of serotonin deficiency are anxiety, insatiable appetite (particularly for carbohydrates), disturbed sleep (difficulty falling to sleep and staying asleep), depression, hopelessness, nervousness, irritability, sexual imbalance and compulsive behavior. Tryptophan is the most effective serotonin producer currently known. Serotonin is also a precursor for melatonin, which has shown to have anti-cancer properties. For nearly half a century L-Tryptophan has been used as a safe and natural alternative to pharmaceutical tranquilizers.

Form: Capsules (500 mg. each)

Suggested Use: One capsule for every 50 pounds of body weight, given in the evening or as directed by a physician. Allow sixty days for full benefit. Best taken without food or with food or beverage that is low in protein. As with any supplement it is recommended to increase dosage slowly. Do not exceed 4 gm (8 capsules) per day.

Available from: BIOS Biochemicals Corp. 1-800-404-8185 or *www.biochemicals.com*

L-Tyrosine This amino acid is also a precursor for the production of a primary thyroid hormone, thyroxine, as well as epinephrine and norepinephrine. L-tyrosine may be of benefit in optimizing thyroid hormonal levels, improving mood, concentration, fatigue, anxiety and depression. Tyrosine is non-controversial, safe in low doses and readily available. Doses of 1500 mg/day have been used to produce norepinephrine, which strengthens heart muscle contractions correcting congestive heart failure. Patients with normal thyroid hormone levels and healthy hearts may experience palpitations, irritability and increase blood pressure with a 1500mg dose.

Form: Capsules (500 mg. each)

Suggested Use: One capsule three times a day on an empty stomach. Best taken first thing in the morning, mid-day and before bedtime.

Available from: ICNR, Inc. order from web site *www.icnr.com* or 1-800-272-2323

Other vitamin and mineral supplements that are beneficial in treating depression are:

- *Inositol:* A relative to glucose that is effective in the treatment of depression as well as panic attacks and mental illness.

   Recommended dosage: four to eight tablets daily in divided doses between meals.

   Available from: ICNR, Inc. order from web site *www.icnr.com* or 1-800-272-2323

- *Magnesium:* Low levels of this mineral heighten nerve impulses that lead to nervous conditions. Supplementing with magnesium can be helpful in cases of depression accompanied by panic attacks or anxiety.

   Recommended dosage: four to six capsules daily in divided doses between meals.

   Available from: ICNR, Inc. order from web site *www.icnr.com* or 1-800-272-2323

- *Natural B-complex vitamins:* This group of vitamins supports normal function of the entire nervous system. Most people do not get enough B-complex vitamins from a daily diet.

   Recommended dosage: four to six tablets daily in divided doses between meals.

   Available from: ICNR, Inc. order from web site *www.icnr.com* or 1-800-272-2323

- *Phosphatidylserine:* This nutritional supplement is effective in alleviating depression.

   Recommended dosage: two to four capsules daily

   Available at Life Extension

   www.inetsupermall.com/life_extension.htm?OVRAW=Life%20Extension&OVKEY= extension%20life&OVMTC=standard

- *SAMe:* It works closely with folic acid and vitamin B-12, and functions as a methyl donor. This nutrient carries and donates methyl molecules necessary to facilitate the manufacture of DNA and brain neurotransmitters. Though researchers still only speculate on precisely how this nutrient eases depression, 39 clinical studies have demonstrated its effectiveness and safety. For example, one study at the University of California at Irvine pitted SAMe against a well-established anti-depressant, desipramine. At the end of four weeks, 62% of the people who took SAMe improved significantly, while only 50% of those who took desipramine experienced comparable results. And a review of research shows that SAMe is just as effective as a class of anti-depressants called tricyclics but with fewer and milder side effects. Psychiatrist Richard Brown and neuropharmacologist Teodoro Bottiglieri, authors of *Stop Depression* Nozu (Putnam, 1999), say that though SAMe can hold its own among even the strongest prescription drugs and works more gently on the body. In comparison to St. John's wort, which may take four to six weeks, it works faster, often in the first week of use.

Recommend dosage for depression: It's best to take SAMe Rx Mood on an empty stomach, 30 minutes before breakfast and 30 minutes before lunch. Two divided doses of appropriate number: 5 to 15 capsules (200mg/cap) 1000 to 3000 mg/daily in the morning and afternoon are effective. All supplements and dosages must be tested to enhance effectiveness. Available from Total Health Discount Vitamins at *www.totaldiscountvitamins.com/Merchant/sameframe.htm*

It is strongly advised that depressed patients be evaluated by their physician for potential pathologic conditions such as an under active thyroid gland, mercury poisoning, toxic bowel, Candida, mold or fungal infections, hypoglycemia or food allergies such as gluten, corn, milk or wheat. Also of prime importance is an assessment by a skilled healer (naturopath, nutritionist, chiropractor or other health care professional) who can test organ systems and the need for supplements. It cannot be emphasized enough, that only supplements that test compatible with each patient's body should be taken.

"We don't receive wisdom; we must discover it for ourselves after a journey that no one can take us or spare us.**"**

Marcel Proust (1871-1922)

Section 8

RECOVERING FROM CANCER

It is well-known that cancer and especially the very aggressive ovarian cancer can recur even with the best of treatments. Recurrence has many causes. Some have been identified, some have not. The more obvious causes focus on the existence of residual cancer cells that were not destroyed by initial therapy. There are other co-related factors that directly influence the reformation of cancer. From a clinical perspective, most recurrences are the result of multiple factors working together. These factors include the presence of:

- toxic heavy metals (mercury, cadmium, arsenic, aluminum, lead, nickel, etc.)
- acid tissue environment (from eating acid forming foods and/or imbalances in the autonomic nervous system-see metabolic typing)
- toxic wastes from intestinal putrefactions (constipation and inadequate digestive enzyme levels result in food rotting in the colon)
- sluggish lymphatic system, which prevents adequate drainage of waste material from normal and cancerous cells
- chemical toxicity (dietary sources such as food additives and environmental such as herbicides, insecticides and pesticides)
- hormone imbalances due to consumption of beef or chicken, which have been injected with steroids and growth hormones
- consumption of soy products, which tend to stimulate estrogen receptors
- ingestion of water stored in soft plastic containers. Bis-phenol A is synthetic estrogen and used in polycarbonate plastics to create pliability. Unfortunately bis-phenol A leaches out from plastic into its contents.
- genetic miasms that alter DNA function.

Doctor Samuel Hahnemann, "Father of Homeopathy", discovered genetic miasms over 200 years ago. He recognized that genetic disease codes could be transferred from as far back as ten generations. This imprinted code could be present without actual clinical disease symptoms but manifest as behavioral traits or chronicity of symptoms. Under conditions of a lowered immune system, psychological distress, acidosis, nutritional deficiencies, heavy metal or chemical toxicity, these genetic influences become part of the equation that alters DNA. This 'disordered state of the internal economy' is referred to as a miasm.

During Hahnemann's initial years of practice, he found that some of his patients would return with the same symptoms he had previously treated. For some unknown reason, these patients were not responding to his best-selected homeopathic remedies. He concluded there must be a deeper, more profound cause to disease other than the obvious symptoms of the patient. Hahnemann discovered three underlying causes to disease, which he named "miasms" meaning "ghost of an illness". These three miasms are the "residues" of disease passed on to us by our ancestors. They are syphilis, gonorrhea, and psora.

Psora means "itch". Many skin and heart problems are related to this miasm. Syphilis and gonorrhea are well-known virulent venereal diseases, which produce a host of mental, emotional, and physical problems. Researchers have also confirmed and treated four additional miasms. They are tuberculosis, cancer, polio, and yama (energy imbalance).

If one of your ancestors had cancer and was treated, with the medicine of choice for their time, the cancer may be destroyed but the miasm would remain and passed on to their children. As they grew older one or more of the children and grandchildren may experience some or all of the symptoms of the cancer miasm. Other manifestations of the cancer miasm are exhaustion, depression, anxiety, feeling excessively obligated or sometimes overwhelmed, and obesity. The miasm's ability to be passed on to the next generation is why entire families have hereditary predispositions to various physical and emotional disorders.

When acquired by descendents miasms do not normally produce the same conditions of the original disease. However, each miasm has an unmistakable influence on the health and vitality of the mind and body, as it tends to drain and deplete the vital force over time. As Hahnemann concluded, they can warp the body's vital force in such a profound way as to create the most debilitating conditions of schizophrenia or rheumatoid arthritis to the mildest hay fever and headaches. The key to successful treatment is to remove the miasms. This creates a powerful and strengthening influence on the mind and body allowing greater happiness, health, and energy.

Syphilis is another primary miasm and is the most destructive of them all. It contributes to rapid weight loss and the deteriorating condition of bone loss. Osteoarthritis is associated with this miasm. Anytime one observes degenerative or deformed conditions of any of the body, bones and blood diseases (hemophilia) or infections, syphilis is involved. Another classic example of its essential nature is the AIDS virus, which is born from this miasm.

Comprehensive cancer treatment must involve use of homeopathic remedies. A homeopathic 1 M (one to a million dilution) tincture of the syphilis miasm, syphilinum, and cancer miasm, carcinosin, effectively help eliminate the genetic codes. Since the probability is high that these miasms have been passed on, it is imperative that all offspring be treated. Clinical experience has shown that one 2 ounce bottle utilizing a 1M strength using a dosage of 10 drops three times a day is adequate for resolution.

RECURRENCE OF CANCER

In May 2003, the first red flag went up. My wife's CA-125 (tumor marker) increased from its low of 15 to 198. This marked the beginning of our second confrontation with reversing cancer. The beginning of June brought a sensation of abdominal fullness and stomach pain. An internal examination by the gynecologic surgeon confirmed the presence of a small mass, which was corroborated by CAT scan. The bad news was the presence of a half-centimeter tumor. The good news was the fact that during the surgical procedure to remove the original mass there were numerous cancerous seeds present in the lining of the pelvic floor. This information confirmed the beneficial effect of just eight treatments with Dr. Morales in Mexico. The quinoxide, ozone and Insulin Potentiation Therapy (IPT) were effective in eliminating the numerous cancerous seeds. To be totally effective IPT must be continued for several months to eradicate all remaining cancer. Since it is difficult to maintain an active dental practice with absentee management, it would have been impossible for us to prolong our stay in Mexico.

Our journey to locate a practitioner to provide the same treatment was fraught with frustration. Obtaining the special extracts from Mexico was not the problem but locating a skilled medical practitioner who had the same equipment and clinical expertise failed. Since time was of the essence, we had to make a decision on our next course of treatment.

An appointment was set up with the original gynecologic surgeon. The option of a second surgery did not exist since the tumor was on the tubes exiting the bladder. The delicate anatomy of this area would have required extensive reconstructive procedures. The doctor also explained to us that the complexity of the surgical treatment and high probability of a poor mechanical result would have resulted in my wife living with an unacceptable physical handicap accompanied by ongoing medical complications. At this point our only logical option was chemotherapy. The good did have several advantages: first, our choice to take the alternative route and approach the cancer by building up the immune system bought us quality time. A regime of eating clean and extensive detoxification and regeneration programs dramatically improved the body's defenses. Second, our delay witnessed a change in the chemotherapeutic agent de jour. The previous combination of paclitaxel plus carboplatin caused horrific side effects. One of the most notable was permanent peripheral nerve damage that manifests as numbness of the hands and feet. As of July 1, 2003, the new drug being touted was Docetaxel. Although the overall toxicity levels are less, the reality is that survival with Docetaxel is no better than with the previous chemotherapeutic agents. Third, the residual tumor was in an accelerated growth spurt, which was more advantageous since chemotherapeutic agents are more effective against actively growing cancer cells. Finally, ovarian cancer is one of the few types of cancer that actually respond to chemotherapy. The other forms that also respond are acute lymphocytic leukemia, Hodgkin's disease, testicular and a handful of rare tumors, mainly present in childhood.

Following the first chemotherapy session in August 2003 the blood analysis (drawn on August 20) exhibited a CA 125 level of 61.8, which was down from the previous month's (July 30th) level of 238. The 176.2 point reduction signified that the Docetaxel was destroying the existing tumor. My wife's second and fourth chemotherapy sessions produced even more dramatic results. The CA 125 level plummeted to 9 and 4.5 respectively. Because of the significant drop in the CA 125 tumor marker the oncologist cancelled the scheduled CAT scan until treatment was completed. Now a continued effort must be made by the patient to continue the daily nutritional protocols to detoxify and support the immune system. In all cases integration of the best of both philosophies must be employed to resolve serious health issues.

Since the health of the immune system is one of the most important factors in any treatment approach to cancer, it is imperative that it is working at its maximum level. One product in the field of immune modulators, MGN-3™, is extracted from rice bran and treated enzymatically with an extract from Shiitake mushrooms. This extract, arabinoxylan, is an effective biological response modifier (BRM) that increases natural killer (NK) cell activity and potentiates the activity of conventional chemotherapeutic agents. Natural killer cells function by first recognizing and then binding to their cell wall. This process requires receptor-to-receptor interaction. Next, the NK cell releases granules, which penetrate the cancer cell and ultimately kill it within five minutes. The NK cell is then free to bind to another cancer cell and repeat the same process. As long as NK cells remain active, the body is able to keep cancer and other diseases under control.

Utilizing immune modulating substances like MGN-3™ is absolutely essential since cancer cells have developed defense mechanisms of their own to help protect them from the body's immune system. Cancer cells know how to fight back in a sort of cell war. Researchers have discovered that cancer cells can destroy white blood cells (WBCs) through the phenomenon of phagocytosis, which enables the cancer cell to literally engulf and then destroy WBCs. Scientists have observed three ways in which cancer cells accomplish this. First, cancer cells can capture WBCs by extending two arms around the body's immune cells. Second, they can develop a cup-shaped opening whereby the WBC is drawn inside. A third way is for the cancer cell to extend a long arm to capture the WBC and finally draw it inside the cancer cell where it is digested. In addition, extensive work by other researchers has shown that cancer cells secrete immune-suppressive substances, which inhibit the function of the body's immune system.

There are many biological response modifier products; however, MGN-3™ has several major advantages over other supplements. The immune-boosting effects of MGN-3™ increase the levels of interferon, a compound produced by the body that inhibits the replication of viruses and it increases the formation of Tumor Necrosis Factors, a group of proteins that help destroy cancer cells. When compared to other biological response modifiers, MGN-3™ studies showed an average increase in natural killer cell function of over 200% — an increase that is more meaningful because it comes from studies on humans. Its biggest plus is the fact that it is nontoxic and has not shown hypo-responsiveness in the four years that patients have been followed. MGN-3™ also outperforms other immune-enhancers by its resistance to hyper-responsiveness. MGN-3™ provides a period of gradual increase, followed by a stabilization of immune system activity at the peak level for as long as therapy is continued. Studies on most biological response modifiers — including pharmaceuticals and natural products — only show a period of increase in immune activity, followed by a period of decline despite continuation of therapy. The efficacy of MGN-3™ equals or surpasses the very best immune-modulating drugs available but, in stark contrast to these, exhibits a complete lack of toxicity.

(MGN-3™ potentiates death receptor-induced apoptosis in cancer cells. M. Ghoneum and S. Gollapudi. Drew Univ. of Medicine and Science, Los Angles, CA; UC Irvine, Division of Basic and Clinical Immunology, Irvine, CA.) The complete research data on MGN-3™ can be reviewed at www.publishedresearch.com/MGN3/MGN3.html

Suggested use for adults: For maximum benefit, follow the MGN-3™ Two-Step Program.

> *Step 1:* Mix contents of 1 packet (1000mg) with warm/cold beverage or food 3 times per day for 3 weeks.
>
> *Step 2:* After 3 weeks, reduce dosage to the maintenance level of 1 packet (1000mg) daily.

For best results, take MGN-3™ two hours before or two hours after taking other supplements. Suggested foods to mix with MGN-3™ powder: yogurt, pudding, hot or cold cereal, and applesauce. MGN-3™ is available from Lane Labs (1-800-LANE-005 or *www.lanelabs.com*)

Combating the adverse side effects of chemotherapeutic agents is a real challenge. Although alternative medicine has shown clinically that taking antioxidant supplements will potentiate the cytotoxic effects of chemotherapeutic agents, there is no universally accepted source for information. Patients must rely on their physician's level of knowledge or seek consultation with other nutritionally oriented health care providers. The following protocol is based on my clinical and personal experience and information gleaned from the scientific literature.

It is intended to guide the patient through this difficult period and help augment whatever protocols have been recommended:

- **CLNZ** It is designed to chelate toxic heavy metals such as mercury, lead, nickel, aluminum and beryllium, as well as some toxic chemicals from the body.

  Ingredients: Dandelion Root; Pfaffia; Cinquefoil; Milk Thistle; Mountain Mahogany; Yucca; Vit. E; Wahoo; RNA/DNA Liver Factors; L-Methionine.

  Recommended dosage: Start with one capsule before bedtime and increase to two after ten days.

  Available from: ICNR, Inc. 1-800-272-2323 or order online at *www.icnr.com*

- **Coffee enemas** The beneficial effect reduces the toxic load on the liver. A special Peruvian coffee bean, blonde blend, is available from S.A. Wilsons in Canada (*www.sawilsons.com*). This bean has a high caffeine content, which opens the portal vein to the liver enabling it to dump accumulated poisons. An enema is recommended before chemotherapy and one following. Reducing the toxic levels help reduce the nausea, vomiting, and fatigue.

- **Fresh prepared green juices** A refreshing and healthful combination includes two Granny Smith apples, one tablespoon of flax oil (Barleans or Arrow Head Mills), two table spoons of ground flax seeds, a small piece of ginger root, one garlic clove, two medium stalks of kale and one dozen pieces of Italian parsley. Chlorophyll is one of the best known detoxifiers, and this combination will help lower toxicity levels, provide adequate fiber to reduce constipation, add omega 3 essential fatty acids to provide antioxidant factors, and supply vital enzymes and minerals. Drink one 8-ounce glass each morning.

- **L-Glutathione (Foodform®)** This company is the only producer of all nature glutathione. This tripeptide amino acid provides sulfur bonds to bind heavy metals and other toxic products in the liver. Because each tablet contains 50mg from a food matrix form, its contents are more bio-available than fractionated synthetic sources.

  As an antioxidant, glutathione is essential for allowing lymphocytes (form of white blood cells) to express their full potential, without being hampered by oxygen radical groups that accumulate during the oxygen-requiring development of the immune response. Glutathione is the major internal antioxidant produced by the cell. Glutathione participates directly in the neutralization of free radicals, reactive oxygen compounds, and maintains exogenous antioxidants such as vitamins C and E in their reduced (active) forms. In addition, through direct conjugation, glutathione plays a role in the *detoxification* of many xenobiotics (foreign compounds) both organic and inorganic. Liver levels of glutathione are drastically reduced by use of chemotherapy and must be replaced to monitor normal functions. Recommended dosage: 2 tablets three times a day between meals.

  Available from: ICNR, Inc. 1-800-272-2323 or order online at *www.icnr.com*

▪ **Alpha-Lipoic Acid** Several qualities distinguish alpha-lipoic acid from other antioxidants; it is a universal metabolic antioxidant; neutralizes free radicals in both the fatty and watery regions of cells, in contrast to vitamin C, which is water-soluble and vitamin E, which is fat-soluble.

The body routinely converts some alpha-lipoic acid to dihydrolipoic acid, which appears to be an even more powerful antioxidant. Both forms of lipoic acid quench peroxynitrite radicals, an especially dangerous type consisting of both oxygen and nitrogen, according to a recent paper in FEBS Letters (Whiteman M, et al., FEBS Letters, 1996; 379: 74-6). Peroxynitrite radicals play a role in the development of atherosclerosis, lung disease, chronic inflammation, and neurological disorders.

Alpha-lipoic acid also plays an important role in the synergism of antioxidants. It directly recycles and extends the metabolic life span of vitamin C, glutathione, and coenzyme Q10, and it indirectly renews vitamin E.

An ideal therapeutic antioxidant would fulfill several criteria. These include: absorption from the diet, conversion in cells and tissues into a usable form, a variety of antioxidant actions (including interactions with other antioxidants) in both membrane and aqueous phases, and low toxicity. Alpha-lipoic acid is unique among natural antioxidants in its ability to fulfill all of these requirements, making it a potentially highly effective therapeutic agent in a number of conditions in which oxidative damage has been implicated." In regards to cancer, alpha-lipoic acid can inhibit the activation of "nuclear factor kappa-B," a protein complex involved in cancer and the progression of AIDS. (Suzuki YJ, et al., Biochemical & Biophysical Research Communications, 1992;189:1709-15). In addition, recent data shows that alpha-lipoic acid increases the cytotoxic effects of Vitamin C toward abnormal cells. Recommended dosage: one tablet (100mg) three times a day with meals. Available from: ICNR, Inc. 1-800-272-2323 or order online at *www.icnr.com*

▪ **CoQ-Zyme 30™** Coenzyme Q10 is also known as ubiquinone. It is a fat-soluble vitamin-like substance present in every cell of the human body and serves as a coenzyme for several of the key enzymatic steps in the production of energy within the cell. It also functions as an antioxidant. It will help prevent blood from clumping and becoming sticky. It also increases the effectiveness of most other drugs and even vitamins. Consult a physician if taking blood thinners, aspirin, or other medications that requires monitoring.

For those patients who have ports for intravenous vitamin/antioxidant and or chemotherapy drugs, use of CoQ10 is highly recommended to maintain blood flow without clumping or clotting. Conventional physicians almost always insist on using Coumadin, which is actually rat poison, to thin the blood and prevent stickiness. It makes no logical sense to introduce another poisonous substance in addition to the chemotherapy when better results can be obtained with a natural substance, which has no side effects.

Contrary to what your doctor tells you CoQ10 has been well documented in hospital studies that show its effectiveness in preventing slugging and clotting of the blood. My wife has had her port in place since January 24, 2003 without any incidents. The real culprit is dietary indiscretions. White refined sugar, hydrogenated fats and refined carbohydrates are major causes of the stickiness of the red blood cells and formation of clots. Eating wholesome foods and taking CoQ10 daily will be one of the best "insurance policies" available.
Recommended dosage: two tablets between meals.
Available from: ICNR, Inc. 1-800-272-2323 or order online at *www.icnr.com*

- **Catalyn®** Derived from organically grown food (carrots, alfalfa, sea vegetables, etc.) this multiple vitamin provides an excellent source of many essential nutrients to maintain normal body function.
  Recommended dosage: three tablets with each meal- chewed.
  Available from: ICNR, Inc. 1-800-272-2323 or order online at *www.icnr.com*

- **Empower C®** Vitamin C is a well-known anti-oxidant that scavenges free radicals and protects against oxidative DNA damage. An anti-oxidant is a chemical that reduces or prevents oxidation, thus preventing cell and tissue damage from free radicals in the body. Since vitamin C is a six-carbon sugar, it is readily absorbed into cancer cells where it inhibits the carcinogenic effects of hydrogen peroxide on intercellular communication. Until this finding, the mechanism for vitamin C's inhibitory effects on carcinogenic tumor formation was not understood. (C.Y. Lee, Cornell professor of food science and technology, and his South Korean colleagues, Ki Won Lee, Hyong Joo Lee and Kyung-Sun Kang, found the connection.)
  Recommended dosage: Three tables (300mg each tablet) three times a day with meals.
  Available from: ICNR, Inc. 1-800-272-2323 or order online at *www.icnr.com*

- **Calcifood Wafers®** This product is produced from raw veal bone and supplies many of the vitamin and nutrients that support the formation of red blood cells and other components.
  Recommended dosage: two tablets three times a day taken between meals and chewed.
  Available from: ICNR, Inc. 1-800-272-2323 or order online at *www.icnr.com*

- **Liver Cleanser Formula** A combination formula effective in detoxification of the liver and boosting the immune system. It contains the following ingredients: amino acids (alanine, arginine, aspartic acid, cysteine, glycine, histidine and tyrosine), Astragalus, cayenne pepper, genseng, glutamic acid milk thistle, saw palmetto berry, shittake mushroom.
  Recommended dosage: two capsules three times a day taken between meals.
  Available from: ICNR, Inc. 1-800-272-2323 or order online at *www.icnr.com*

- **Optygen**™ The primary component of Optygen™ is Rhodiola rosea (Golden root). This herb has pharmacological properties as an anti-mutagen and *anti-depressive agent*. But Rhodiola rosea is much more powerful than other adaptogens. In one study by O.M. Duhan and colleagues, the anti-mutagenic activities of Panax Ginseng and of Rhodiola rosea were compared. The extracts of Rhodiola rosea had a higher capacity to counteract gene mutations induced by various mutagens (up to about 90% inhibition in some cases). The *anti-depressive and anti-stress activity* of Golden root is higher than St. John's Wort, Ginkgo biloba and Panax Ginseng.

  Recommended dosage: One capsule three times a day between meals. Some patients may require an initial dose twice the recommended to support their weakened adrenal glands.

  Available from: ICNR, Inc. 1-800-272-2323 or order online at *www.icnr.com*

- **Sesame Oil** This oil provides all the essential amino acids, especially methionine and tryptophan. Methionine is high in sulfur, which detoxifies heavy metals and other toxic wastes. Tryptophan is the precursor for serotonin, a neurotransmitter that imparts the feeling of well-being and niacin, which is essential for nerve function. Sesame oil contains large amounts of thiamin (B-1) Riboflavon (B-2) and Niacin (B-3), nutrients that support the normal function of the nervous system. Also present is a fraction, which is sometimes referred to as vitamin T, which the FDA does not recognize, but is valuable in supporting the immune system. When taken with Thymex®, the combination boosts the immune system helping to prevent and or fight infections.

  Recommended dosage: one perle three times a day between meals.

  Available from: ICNR, Inc. 1-800-272-2323 or order online at *www.icnr.com*

- **Thymex®** A protomorphagen, it is derived from bovine thymus tissue. Protomorphagens provide the genetic blue print for tissue repair. Although the thymus gland shrinks in size around puberty, it still functions to support the body's immune system. The thymus gland aids in the production of antibodies, which react against foreign protein. The vitality of this organ is essential to help fight off infections. Thymex® is one of the critical immune boosters essential in resolving hepatitis C.

  Recommended dosage: two tablets three times a day taken between meals.

  Available from: ICNR, Inc. 1-800-272-2323 or order online at *www.icnr.com*

END OF A JOURNEY

Reversing cancer is not an easy journey. Mistakes will be made along the way. Hopefully they will be minor and lessons will be learned. Most patients panic when they are given a diagnosis of cancer. It is during this period of distress and uncertainty that they are most vulnerable and easily intimidated by spouses, children, friends and well meaning but misinformed physicians. Most patients have been conditioned by the medical establishment to present their body to be healed. This is not how it works. A team approach is essential to combine the best of both schools, taking what conventional medicine and alternative medicine have to offer and formulating a plan. In addition, one must also do their own research to find out what is available and which practitioners have the best clinical skills to administer the treatment. One must also take an active part in changing their lifestyle (food intake, exercise and spirituality). Do not be afraid to express ideas. Even without a medical degree common sense combined with reading books, articles and information from consultant reports regarding cancer will permit a more intelligent discussion of options. If a physician is not willing to be open-minded and help you explore options, find a new doctor. Interview the next physician to determine in advance their philosophy of healing. Unfortunately most people spend more time planning a surprise birthday party for their spouse than they do in researching cancer treatment and prospective physicians. Planning ahead will result in fewer problems and issues during therapy.

Sacrifices in both time and money will have to be made to achieve remission and in some cases a cure. Reversing Cancer was written as a result of our own healing journey. It is hoped that our experiences and knowledge will make it easier for cancer patients to have a better overall understanding of the nature of cancer, the alternative treatments available and choices of effective nutrients. Having this invaluable information in one source will make your own journey easier, more economical, faster and less fearful. The journey can be an exciting adventure with new challenges. In the end the patient must be comfortable with making the best, informed decisions.

May the healing journey be a peaceful one.

Appendices

Appendix I

SUPPLEMENT SCHEDULE

Upon Awakening

- 1 tsp Aloe Vera
- 2 ounces detox tea (plus 2 oz. water)
- 1 Cats Claw
- 2 Q-Max + 2 Co Q- Zyme 30
- 2 MSM

- 8 drops Hydroxygen
- 2 ounces fresh wheatgrass juice
- 1 Boswellia complex
- 1 Artemisinin
- 2 Transfer Factor Plus

Breakfast

- 3 Cyruta Plus (vitamin C)
- 1 Black Currant Seed Oil
- 2 Catalyn (general multiple)
- 1 Formula 1 (rebalance ANS*)

- 2 Lipoic acid
- 2 Quercetin
- 3 Cataplex B (stimulates ANS)
- 2 Perfect Food (general multiple + enzymes)

Between Meals

- 3 Grape PiPs
- 4 ProactEnz
- 2 Transfer Factor Plus
- 2 ounces detox tea (plus 2 oz. water)

- 8 Drops Hydroxygen
- 2 Q-Max + 2 Co Q-Zyme 30
- 1 Artemisinin

Lunch

- 3 Cyruta Plus (vitamin C)
- 1 Black Currant Seed Oil
- 2 Catalyn (general multiple)
- 1 Formula 1 (rebalance ANS)

- 2 Lipoic acid
- 2 Quercetin
- 3 Cataplex B (stimulates ANS)
- 2 Perfect Food (general multiple + enzymes)

Between Meals

- 3 Grape PiPs
- 4 ProactEnz
- 2 Transfer Factor Plus
- 2 ounces detox tea (plus 2 oz. water)

- 8 Drops Hydroxygen
- 2 Q-Max + 2 Co Q-Zyme 30
- 1 Artemisinin

Dinner

- 3 Cyruta Plus (vitamin C)
- 1 Black Currant Seed Oil
- 2 Catalyn (general multiple)
- 1 Formula 1 (rebalance ANS)

- 2 Lipoic acid
- 2 Quercetin
- 3 Cataplex B (stimulates ANS)
- 2 Perfect Food (general multiple + enzymes)

Bedtime

- 8 drops Hydroxygen
- 2 ounces detox tea (plus 2 oz. water)
- Coffee enema (Blond Blend- 2 cups)
- 1 Tbs Bulgaricum (probiotic) + water
- 1 Glutathione

- 1 CLNZ
- 4 ProactEnz
- 1 Garlic tablet (2000 mg)
- 1 Boswellia complex
- Transfer Factor

This supplement schedule was custom designed and tested for patient compatibility; using this program on all patients does not guarantee results.

Appendix II

TUMOR MARKERS — STAGE III OVARIAN CANCER

Test Dates	CA 125*	LASA-P**
Prior to surgery	840	N/A
Dec. 9, 2002: Date of surgery		
Dec. 23, 2002: Rife Tx	130	N/A
Jan. 7, 2003: Nutrition	32	24
Feb. 4, 2003: Detoxification	32	17.2
Mar. 5, 2003: IPT + Oxidative Tx	15	17.5
IPT therapy reduced the CA 125 by 50%		
May 2003	198	None
July 30, 2003	238	None
Chemotherapy started August 1, 2003		
August 20, 2003	61.8	None
September 11, 2003	9	None
October 3, 2003	4.7	None
October 22, 2003	4.5	None
October 24, 2003	3.2	None
November 10, 2003	2.5	None
February 6, 2004	2.2	None
Normal Range	**0-20 U/mL**	**15-20 mg/dL**

*Cancer Antigen, **Lipid Associated Sialic Acid in Plasma (LASA-P)

CAT SCAN EVALUATION OF ABDOMINAL REGION

December 17, 2003	No visible sign of metastasis or existing tumor.

Appendix III

The following information is supplied to answer most of the questions that prospective cancer patients have about IPT treatment.

Who is the ideal candidate for IPT:
- Patients with newly diagnosed cancer
- Tumor load small (ideal after surgical removal of tumor)
- No metastases (positive results have been achieved with metastases)
- No previous treatment (chemotherapy damages the immune system and decreases success rate)
- No concomitant medical conditions

For the person with the above criteria, the likelihood of success with IPT is strong. It doesn't mean that someone who has, had, previous chemotherapy, has multiple medical conditions, or has a high tumor load should not try IPT, but the prognosis isn't as positive as when the above criteria are met and that the amount of treatments and medications used may need to be increased. Even in medically compromised patients success can be achieved with a comprehensive nutritional program.

How Many IPT Treatments Will Be Needed? Most cancers are evaluated after six to ten IPT treatments. Generally, IPT is utilized to treat a cancer until one of the following responses occurs:
- Cancer goes into remission
- Cancer is arrested
- IPT clearly is not working

If after six or ten treatments of IPT there has been no tumor regression, the treatment regime is either stopped or changed. IPT is a flexible treatment. The regime can be changed, and often it is to decrease the chance of drug resistance. IPT helps enhance the effects of chemotherapy (synthetic or naturally derived) medications but still depends on the particular cancer being sensitive to the chemotherapeutic agent(s) being used.

The total number of treatments needed often depends on the aggressiveness and rapidity of growth of the cancer. For the person with a newly diagnosed rapidly growing cancer (cancer popped up with a month or two) the response with IPT is often quite rapid, within the first round of IPT treatments. For someone with a more indolent type of cancer that is slow growing, the number of treatments typically will be more. Implementing a detoxification and nutritional program will greatly enhance the effectiveness of IPT.

Two coffee enemas are strongly recommended on the days that IPT treatment is given. This will greatly reduce the toxic burden on the liver and immune system and reduce the number of IPT sessions required to resolve the cancer. It is impossible to know how many IPT treatments a patient will need. But if the tumor is shrinking with IPT, do not take a break from IPT! While a tumor is being destroyed, it is imperative to enhance the immune system with nutrients. Making the body more alkaline and oxygenating the tissues will further help to destroy the cancer. Tumors have a tremendous resiliency, but improving the health of the tissues of the body will decrease the cancer's ability to survive. To insure long-term success, lifestyles must be altered or else the same conditions that set the stage for the cancer will cause it to return! Tumors can build up drug resistance. This can be overcome by using Rife technology because cancer cells do not become resistant to frequencies. It is imperative that adjunctive therapy aimed at strengthening the immune system, and increasing the oxygenation of tissues and fluid be continued. A multi-therapy approach with goals tailored to the patient's needs will be the most successful.

How Often Do I Need to Get IPT? The success of IPT depends upon its ability to kill more cancer cells between each treatment than will be replicated. Between IPT treatments there is always the risk that cancer cells will replicate and grow, so IPT is generally given at least weekly. Some people need more frequent treatments as often as twice to three times a week. Use of Rife frequencies between IPT treatments will greatly reduce the number of cancer cells and enhance IPT.

How Long Do I Have To Fast Before IPT? IPT treatment works best when the patient does not eat the day of treatment. Ideally the patient should fast overnight before getting IPT. Patients can drink water in the morning of the treatment but nothing else. Medications or herbs should not be taken on the day of treatment unless they have been approved in advance. Patients who receive IPT in the afternoon, must fast at least four hours before treatment.

How Will I Feel During IPT? IPT is predicated on the fact that insulin opens up the membranes surrounding cells to help them feed by increasing their glucose concentration. This decreases the blood sugar level and induces a hypoglycemic reaction. Typical symptoms include, fatigue, mental fog, shaky, rapid heart rate, (sweaty and warm and/or cold). Each patient will experience these symptoms when their blood sugar levels fall within a range of 40 to 50. The on set of severe symptoms signifies a therapeutic window. Within the next 30 minutes the natural or synthetic chemotherapeutic agent is given.

   Once the chemotherapeutic agents are given, the person is then given Gatoraid®, power or fruit drinks to reverse the hypoglycemic symptoms. Within a few minutes, they feel relief.

Can Adjunctive Treatments Be Given? Adjunctive therapy is encouraged. Additional treatment in tandem with IPT can include photo luminescent agents and Quinoxide. Once these substances are given intravenously, the patient's blood can be withdrawn, placed in a glass bottle and mixed with ozone. The blood is then run through a special quartz tube and exposed to infra red and ultraviolet frequencies and returned to the patient via the intravenous line. Approximately 15 minutes of additional light therapy (infrared and laser) is then applied over the area of the cancer.

On the days between IPT treatments, patients are encouraged to get intravenous drips of vitamins, hydrogen peroxide or quinoxide. These treatments help bolster the immune system and kill cancer cells.

Can I Eat After IPT? The patient must bring a salad and or sandwiches for immediate consumption following the infusion of the chemotherapeutic agents. A normal evening meal can be eaten. IPT is generally very well tolerated. Patients who reduce their overall toxicity levels prior to IPT treatment have minimal or no side effects. The key is to commence the detoxification program as soon as possible after the diagnosis and before IPT.

How Low Does The Blood Sugar Go With IPT? Typically during IPT the blood sugar drops to between 20 and 40. Normal blood sugar is between 75 and 110. Because individual responses to insulin vary, it may take a few visits to get the blood sugar to drop that low.

Are There Any Side Effects To IPT? As of February 2001, Dr. Donato Perez Garcia's three generations of family physicians provided IPT treatment for a combined total of 102 years. Their total morbidity for three generations of IPT treatment was zero. In comparison, 300,000 patients die each year in conventional hospitals from common mistakes.

- Donato Perez Garcia, Sr., M.D. (ORIGINATOR OF IPT) (1896-1971)
  YEARS OF DOING IPT 1930-1971: 41 YEARS MORTALITY 0%
- Donato Perez Garcia Bellon, M.D. (1930-2000)
  YEARS OF DOING IPT 1956-2000: 44 YEARS MORTALITY 0%
- Donato Perez Garcia, Jr., M.D. (Still living)
  YEARS OF DOING IPT 1983-2000: 17 YEARS MORTALITY 0%

The group of physicians who founded IPT and have over 100 years of experience with it, have never had a person die because of IPT. Because the doses of chemotherapy medications used during IPT are 10-25% of the amounts given during traditional cancer care, the risk of side effects is greatly diminished. The most common side effect from IPT is fatigue during the day of treatment. Nausea occurs only rarely.

IPT is a viable alternative to high dose chemotherapy with all of its side effects, which can include immunosuppression, hair loss, nerve, heart, kidney, and liver damage. IPT can also cause these side effects, but they are almost non-existent because of the low dose of medications used.

Are There Any Absolute Contraindications to IPT? There are no absolute contraindications to IPT. There are factors that can interfere with a person's response to IPT such as previous chemotherapy, radiation therapy, poor immune function, and hopelessness, but again, these do not preclude someone from having IPT. Remember where there is life there is hope.

Can I Take Supplements While Undergoing IPT? True comprehensive natural medicine care for cancer involves potent nutraceutical supplementation. Appropriate nutritional supplementation during IPT can have multiple beneficial effects including immune stimulation, liver detoxification, protection of normal cells against chemotherapy, and potentiation of the chemotherapy effect on the cancer cells. Nutritional supplementation is a vital part of any cancer treatment protocol, *however, it is imperative that all supplements be tested for each patient instead of shot gunning a mass of products.*

Who Can do IPT? IPT can be done by any licensed physician. But be aware that most physicians are not trained in IPT. Be sure to seek out a physician experienced in IPT treatment.

Recommended Clinic for IPT Treatment:

Rio Valley Medical Center
Dr. Frank J. Morales, Jr.
Ave. Alvaro Obregon #77
Matamoros, Tamps.
01152 (86) 8812-48-42

U.S.A. Telephone Number: 1-956-592-5586
Fax: 1-956-544-4439
email: frankstaf@hotmail.com

U

V

W

X

Z